ONCOLOGY

FOR MEDICAL STUDENTS
AND JUNIOR DOCTORS

Dr Matthew Langtree

Dr Ning Ma

Published in the United Kingdom by

Stafford Books

Email: info@staffordbooks.co.uk

First printed December 2013

ISBN 978-0957156333

Medical knowledge is always changing. New research and developments happen every day. Readers are advised that the most appropriate management may frequently change and as such it is the practitioners responsibility to ensure that current advice is sought when appropriate. Neither the author nor publisher assume any liability for any injury or damage arising from the information contained within this book. If however, you do notice any errors or have any suggestions for future editions, the author can be contacted by e-mail: support@staffordbooks.co.uk

Stafford books would like to credit the following sources for some of the photographs used in this book:
National Cancer Institute
Dr. Lance Liotta Laboratory
Skin Cancer Foundation

For Frank, Aiping, Nigel and Joe

CONTENTS

CONTENTS

COLORECTAL CANCER

EPIDEMIOLOGY

- Colorectal cancer is the third most common cancer in the UK (13% of diagnoses)
- It is the second most common cause of cancer death in the UK
- Three-quarters of those diagnosed are aged over 65
- 7% of cases are familial
- Colon cancer is equally as common in males and females, but rectal cancer is more common in males

RISK FACTORS INCLUDE

- Family history of colorectal cancer
- Hereditary nonpolyposis colorectal cancer (HNPCC)
- Polyposis syndromes such as familial adenomatous polyposis, Gardner syndrome and Peutz-Jeghers syndrome
- Colorectal disease such as previous colorectal cancer, previous small bowel cancer, inflammatory bowel disease (especially ulcerative colitis) and cholecystectomy
- High intake of red meat and animal fat
- Low intake of fibre, folate and calcium
- Sedentary lifestyle and obesity
- Smoking and high alcohol intake
- There is also evidence for diabetes mellitus, hormonal factors (oestrogen related), certain occupational hazards (particularly asbestos) and renal transplantation with its associated immunosuppression
- There is good evidence that low dose daily aspirin (and other NSAIDs) reduce the risk by 20-40% and 30 minutes of exercise a day reduces risk by a quarter

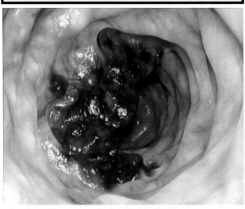

A malignant tumour growing into the intestinal lumen

SIGNS & SYMPTOMS

Right sided
- Anaemia (microcytic)
- Occult bleeding
- Weight loss
- Palpable right iliac fossa mass

Right sided tumours are more likely to be advanced at presentation than left sided tumours and therefore features such as ascites or hepatomegaly are more common

Left sided
- Altered bowel habit
- Tenesmus
- Rectal bleeding
- Colicky pain
- Mass

As an emergency
- Occasionally patients can present with intestinal obstruction or peritonitis

Rectal tumour
- The main features of a rectal tumour are bleeding and irritation

INVESTIGATIONS

- PR examination
- Bloods including LFTs and CEA
- Proctoscopy
- Sigmoidoscopy
- Colonoscopy +/- barium enema
- Endoscopic biopsy
- CT colonoscopy
- CT scan for staging
- MRI or endorectal ultrasound for local extent of rectal tumour
- Liver imaging (ultrasound or MRI)
- PET scan, particularly in recurrence

STAGING AND PROGNOSIS

- The Dukes' staging system is used
A – Confined to mucosa and submucosa
B – Penetrated muscularis mucosa
C – Regional lymph node involvement
D – Distant metastasis
- TNM staging is also used
- Overall five year survival is 50%
- Median survival for untreated metastatic disease is 6-8 months
- But survival rates in the UK are improving

COLORECTAL CANCER

TREATMENT OPTIONS

- Multidisciplinary team discussion
- Surgery remains the first choice therapy
- TMR (total mesorectal excision) has become the main surgery for rectal tumours and other commonly performed surgeries include sigmoid, left or right hemicolectomies and anterior resection
- Large randomised control trials have shown survival benefits of adjuvant 5-fluorouracil or capecitabine chemotherapy in patients with lymph node involvement
- FOLFOX, the addition of oxaliplatin (and folinic acid) further improves survival (but side effects include peripheral neuropathy)
- FOLFIRI is an alternative (irinotecan instead of oxaliplatin), but side effects include hair loss
- These chemotherapy agents can also prolong survival of advanced metastatic disease by around 6-12 months
- Radiotherapy is not routinely used for colon tumours, but has a role for rectal disease
- Radiotherapy reduces the incidence of recurrence of rectal tumours which has a greater impact upon mortality than metastatic disease
- Monoclonal antibodies such as cetuximab can have a role in metastatic disease
- Liver resection is only possible in around a quarter of cases of liver metastasis

SCREENING/TYPES/ PATHOLOGY

- 98% of tumours are adenocarcinomas with 20% being mucinous in type
- The tumour may be nodular, ulcerating or polypoid in appearance
- One-third of tumours occur in the rectum, and the rest in the colon
- The main (and first) site of metastasis is the liver, but spread can also occur to the lungs, brain and bone
- CEA has no role in initial screening, but can be helpful in follow up to help detect recurrence
- In the UK, faecal occult blood test kits are offered on a two yearly basis to individuals between the ages of 60 and 74 as a method of screening
- Those that have moderate or high risk of disease are offered colonoscopies at regular intervals

OTHER INTERESTING POINTS

- Around 15% of patients with unresectable liver metastases at initial presentation can become resectable if they respond well to chemotherapy

KEY POINTS SUMMARY

- Colorectal cancer is the third most common malignancy and the second leading cause of cancer death in the UK
- Advancing age, family history and inflammatory bowel disease are the key risk factors
- There is good evidence that aspirin has a protective effect
- Faecal occult blood testing is used as a screening method
- Two thirds of tumours occur in the colon and the remainder in the rectum
- Colorectal cancer tends to present in one of three ways; asymptomatic individuals detected by screening, with chronic symptoms or as an emergency admission
- Colonoscopy is the gold standard investigation in symptomatic individuals as it also allows biopsies to be taken
- Surgery is the primary treatment in fit individuals as this is the only potential for cure
- CEA levels should be measured before surgery as it can have a role in follow up for detecting potential recurrence
- 20% of patients will have metastatic disease at diagnosis
- Most patients that present with metastatic disease are not appropriate candidates for curative surgical procedures
- Adjuvant chemotherapy is recommended post potentially curative surgery as this improves cure rates, particularly in those with stage III (node positive) disease
- TNM or Dukes' staging can be used and this is the best predictive factor for survival
- Overall five year survival is 50%

OESOPHAGEAL CANCER

EPIDEMIOLOGY

- Oesophageal carcinoma is the eighth most common cancer in the UK
- It is the leading cause of cancer death in China
- It is more common in males
- Incidence increases rapidly in those aged over 55
- Incidence rates in the UK are considerably higher than the European average

RISK FACTORS INCLUDE

- Excess alcohol
- Smoking
- Barrett's Oesophagus/reflux disease
- Nutritional deficiencies (particularly vitamin A, vitamin C, riboflavin and zinc)
- Patterson-Brown-Kelly syndrome
- Obesity
- Achalasia
- Oesophageal stasis from any other cause
- Tylosis
- Occupation (particularly the rubber industry)

SIGNS & SYMPTOMS

- Dysphagia
- Odynophagia
- Weight loss
- Regurgitation
- Retrosternal pain/dyspepsia
- Cough
- Hoarse voice
- Lymphadenopathy
- Symptoms of gastrointestinal blood loss such as melaena or those from anaemia

INVESTIGATIONS

- Endoscopy (with biopsy)
- Double contrast barium swallow (to demonstrate tumour length)
- Endoluminal ultrasound (for tumour depth)
- Staging CT scan
- Blood tests including FBC, LFTs, U&Es, CRP and glucose
- Also consider an FNAC of any lymph nodes, a chest x-ray and bronchoscopy in suspected tracheal involvement and a PET scan to help select surgical candidates

TYPES/PATHOLOGY/ SCREENING

- Upper third (10%) and middle third (40%) tumours are usually squamous cell carcinomas (SCC)
- Lower third tumours (50%) are usually adenocarcinomas arising from glandular metaplastic mucosa (Barrett's Oesophagus)

TREATMENT OPTIONS

- Multidisciplinary team discussion
- One third of patients are suitable for surgery, which has better overall outcomes, but in reality the prognosis remains poor
- The Mckeown procedure (for upper third tumours) and the Ivor Lewis procedure (for middle and lower third tumours) are examples of surgical options
- Chemotherapy (cisplatin and 5-flurouracil) or chemoradiation is a common component of radical treatment
- For non-operable tumours, treatment is mostly palliative
- Palliative options include stent insertion, radiotherapy, chemotherapy, laser therapy or a combination of these
- Nutritional support including nasogastric tubes and PEG or RIG insertion
- Symptom control

STAGING & PROGNOSIS

- The TNM system is used
- In the UK, five year survival is less than 10% for non-resectable disease
- Due to longitudinal spread and early spread to surrounding structures five year survival rates following surgery remain poor (20%)

OTHER INTERESTING POINTS

- Helicobacter pylori infection can reduce the risk of developing oesophageal cancer
- NSAIDs and aspirin use may also reduce the risk
- Over the last twenty years the incidence of SCC has remained static, whilst the incidence of adenocarcinoma has been increasing
- The high incidence rate in China and Iran has been linked to food preservatives

GASTRIC CANCER

EPIDEMIOLOGY

- Gastric cancer is the fourth most common cancer worldwide (and leading cause of cancer death in Japan), but only the sixth most common cancer in the UK
- It is more common in males, those aged over 60 and those in lower socioeconomic groups

RISK FACTORS INCLUDE

- Helicobacter Pylori infection
- Diet (salt and nitrates and low intake of fresh fruit and vegetables)
- Deficiency of selenium and vitamins A, C & E
- Blood group A
- Atrophic gastritis
- Achlorhydria
- Pernicious anaemia
- Familial risk
- Hypogammaglobulinaemia

SIGNS & SYMPTOMS

- Dysphagia
- Dyspepsia
- Vomiting
- Weight loss
- Abdominal pain
- Sensation of epigastric fullness
- Epigastric mass
- Symptoms of anaemia
- Troisier's sign, which is an enlarged left supraclavicular node (Virchow's node)

TYPES/PATHOLOGY/ SCREENING

- 95% are adenocarcinoma
- Half of all tumours occur in the pyloric region and a further quarter occur on the lesser curve
- Metastatic spread can occur directly to adjacent structures, lymphatically (via celiac nodes), transcoelomically (peritoneal seedlings and Krukenberg tumours of the ovaries) and heamatogenously (via the portal or systemic systems)
- Endoscopic screening programmes have been introduced in countries which have a very high incidence, such as Japan and Korea
- Early detection and excellent results from gastrectomy with extensive lymph node resection have led to a better five year survival

INVESTIGATIONS

- Routine blood tests
- Endoscopy and biopsy
- Barium meal
- CT for staging
- Endoscopic ultrasound for tumour depth
- Laparoscopy

TREATMENT OPTIONS

- Multidisciplinary team discussion
- Surgery is the only potentially curative treatment modality
- Surgery is possible in around 75% of patients in the UK
- Partial or total gastrectomy is the most commonly performed surgery
- Combined neoadjuvant and adjuvant chemotherapy has been shown to increase survival
- Stand alone adjuvant treatment, which is not standard treatment in the UK does not appear to be so beneficial
- 5-flurouricil is the most effective chemotherapy agent, and is often combined with other agents such as epirubicin and cisplatin (ECF regime)
- Radiotherapy can be of benefit as an adjuvant to surgery, but its role in palliative care is limited by side effects (the exception is when there is bleeding from tumours) or for bone metastases
- Palliative chemotherapy has been shown to produce survival and quality of life benefit
- Palliative surgery and endoscopic procedures such as stents and laser coagulation should also be considered
- Nutritional needs and support should also be addressed

STAGING & PROGNOSIS

- The TNM system is used
- There is a 20% overall five year survival

OTHER INTERESTING POINTS

- Over the last few decades, the proportion of gastric carcinoma in the cardia has been increasing, whilst that in the pyloric region has been decreasing

HEPATOCELLULAR CANCER

EPIDEMIOLOGY

- Hepatocellular carcinoma is the most common type of primary liver cancer
- It is rare in the UK, but common in sub-Saharan Africa and Asia
- The average age of diagnosis in the UK is 66
- It is much more common in males

RISK FACTORS INCLUDE

- Hepatitis B
- Hepatitis C
- Alcoholic cirrhosis
- Haemochromatosis
- Chronic autoimmune hepatitis
- Aflatoxin (from Aspergillus fungus in mouldy food)
- Alpha-1 antitrypsin deficiency
- Primary biliary sclerosis
- Wilson's disease
- Metabolic syndrome, diabetes and smoking

SIGNS & SYMPTOMS

- Right upper quadrant abdominal pain
- Weight loss
- Jaundice
- Ascites
- Pruritus
- Hepatomegaly
- Splenomegaly (and oesophageal varices, especially if portal vein thrombosis occurs)
- Arterial bruit and hepatic rub over the tumour
- Hypoglycaemia (from insulin like peptide secretion)
- Hypercalcaemia (from PTH secretion)
- Feminisation (from oestrogen secretion)

INVESTIGATIONS

- Routine blood tests including a clotting screen
- Serum alpha-fetoprotein
- Hepatitis screen
- Abdominal ultrasound
- Staging CT scan
- Angiography, MRI and doppler flow studies can provide useful information
- Core biopsy or FNAC (under radiological guidance)

TYPES/PATHOLOGY/SCREENING

- Hepatocellular carcinoma tends to occur from regenerating nodules in a cirrhotic liver
- They can be multifocal and intrahepatic spread is common
- The lungs and bone are the most common sites of systemic metastatic spread

TREATMENT OPTIONS

- Multidisciplinary team discussion
- Surgical resection is the mainstay of radical treatment, but is only possible in 10-15%
- Liver transplantation may be suitable in carefully selected patients (the Milan criteria can help)
- Alternative options include hepatic artery embolisation, intravenous chemotherapy, intra-hepatic artery chemotherapy, interferon alpha, percutaneous ethanol injection (for small tumours), radiofrequency ablation and microwave ablation
- Hepatocellular carcinoma is relatively chemoresistant to systemic chemotherapy
- There is some growing evidence for the use of molecular targeted therapies such as sorafenib
- There is little role for radiotherapy, even in palliation

STAGING AND PROGNOSIS

- A number of staging systems have been developed including the Cancer of the Liver Italian Program (CLIP) and the Barcelona Clinic Liver Cancer (BCLC) staging and treatment approach
- Overall survival is 3% at five years (25% survival in successfully resected disease)

OTHER INTERESTING POINTS

- Hepatocellular carcinoma is the sixth most commonly occurring cancer worldwide
- The incidence is so high in parts of Africa and Asia due to hepatitis B being epidemic
- Alpha-fetoprotein is raised in 80% of presentations, but may also be elevated in germ cell tumours, liver metastases from the stomach or pancreas and mildly so in viral hepatitis and active cirrhosis

PANCREATIC CANCER

EPIDEMIOLOGY

- Pancreatic cancer is the fifth most common cause of cancer death in the UK, whilst only being the eleventh most common cancer overall
- It predominantly occurs in the seventh and eighth decades of life
- Incidence rates are similar for males and females

RISK FACTORS INCLUDE

- Smoking
- Alcohol
- Diet high in animal fats
- Obesity
- Chronic pancreatitis
- Diabetes mellitus (especially late onset)
- Gastric ulceration (especially those who have had surgery)
- Inflammatory bowel disease
- Family history of pancreatic cancer
- Some familial cancer syndromes

SIGNS & SYMPTOMS

- Early symptoms are often vague and non-specific
- Jaundice
- Weight loss
- Back pain
- Abdominal pain
- Fatigue
- Steatorrhoea (malabsorption)
- Thrombophlebitis/thromboembolism
- Palpable gallbladder/Courvoisier's sign
- Upper abdominal mass (late sign)

TYPES/PATHOLOGY/ SCREENING

- 90% are adenocarcinoma
- 80% are ductal adenocarcinoma
- Other types of primary pancreatic tumour include adenosquamous carcinoma, acinar cell carcinoma, giant cell carcinoma and pancreatoblastoma
- 75% occur in the head, 15% in the body and 10% in the tail of the pancreas
- Metastases most commonly occur in the liver, peritoneum and lungs

INVESTIGATIONS

- Blood tests including FBC, LFTs, and glucose
- CA19.9 has a sensitivity of 80% and specificity of 73% for pancreatic cancer. Its main role is in assessing response to treatment and post treatment surveillance
- Abdominal ultrasound scan
- CT scan
- ERCP (or occasionally MRCP)
- Endoscopic ultrasound (EUS) is becoming increasingly important as it is more sensitive than a CT scan and can guide an FNAC

TREATMENT OPTIONS

- Multidisciplinary team discussion
- Surgery is the only potentially curative modality
- Unfortunately only 15% of patients have surgically resectable disease at diagnosis
- The most commonly performed surgery is the Whipple procedure
- Adjuvant chemotherapy (usually 5-fluorouracil or gemcitabine) is recommended as it confers a survival benefit
- Adjuvant radiotherapy with chemotherapy may be of benefit in selected patients
- Unresectable disease tends to be resistant to chemotherapy
- Palliative approaches include surgical bypass or endoscopic stenting for an obstructed biliary tract or duodenal obstruction, pain control that may require a celiac plexus block, pancreatic enzyme supplements for malabsorption and prokinetic antiemetics for nausea and vomiting

STAGING AND PROGNOSIS

- The TNM staging system is used
- Overall five year survival is 4%, but improves to 15-20% for surgically resectable disease

OTHER INTERESTING POINTS

- 10% of patients develop diabetes mellitus
- 5% of the population lack the Lewis (a) antigen and therefore do not produce CA19.9, meaning a negative result does not exclude pancreatic cancer

OTHERS

ANAL CANCER

- Anal cancer is rare and more common in females
- Risk factors include human papillomavirus, immunosuppression (particularly HIV), other sexually transmitted infections, receptive anal intercourse and smoking
- 80% are squamous cell carcinoma and other types include adenocarcinoma, melanoma and lymphoma
- It most frequently presents with anal discomfort or bleeding, but may also present with faecal incontinence, fistulae and lymphadenopathy
- Investigations include PR examination, examination under anaesthetic with biopsy, FNAC of enlarged nodes, endoanal ultrasound, CT, MRI and tests for the relevant predisposing infections
- Combination radiotherapy and chemotherapy is the primary treatment
- Surgery is reserved for those who do not respond or relapse
- Biopsy is important to differentiate an anal tumour from a down growing rectal tumour as the management is different
- The TNM staging system is used
- Five year survival is 60%
- Anal margin tumours have a better prognosis

SMALL BOWEL CARCINOMA

- Small bowel carcinoma accounts for 2% of all gastrointestinal malignancies
- Other small bowel malignancies include carcinoids, lymphomas and sarcomas
- It most commonly affects the duodenum and proximal jejunum
- Pre-existing bowel conditions predispose
- Signs and symptoms include diarrhoea, abdominal pain, nausea, vomiting, mass, anaemia, weight loss and jaundice
- Investigations include barium meal, endoscopy (OGD +/- capsule endoscopy) with biopsy, chest x-ray and abdominal ultrasound or CT
- Surgery is the mainstay of treatment
- Radiotherapy and chemotherapy are not useful in this setting
- Prognosis is poor as disease is often advanced at the time of diagnosis
- Overall five year survival is 35% for duodenal tumours and 20% for tumours in the jejunum

CHOLANGIOCARCINOMA

- Cholangiocarcinoma refers to a carcinoma affecting any part of the biliary tree
- Most cases occur between the ages of 60 and 80 and it is more common in Asia than the UK
- Risk factors include gallstones, sclerosing cholangitis in ulcerative colitis patients, liver flukes, choledochal cysts and some occupational exposures
- More than 90% are adenocarcinomas
- Signs and symptoms include jaundice, hepatomegaly, abdominal pain and pruritus
- Investigations include blood tests, ultrasound, CT, MRI cholangiography and angiography
- Surgical resection is the primary treatment
- Prognosis is poor

GALLBLADDER CANCER

- More common in males and those aged 60-80
- Most (85%) are adenocarcinomas
- Risk factors include gallstones, cholecystitis, polyps, congenital bile duct abnormalities, 'porcelain' gallbladder, family history, smoking and obesity
- Patients may be asymptomatic with the tumour found incidentally at cholecystectomy
- Or it may present with pain, jaundice, weight loss, nausea and vomiting, and abdominal distension
- Investigations include blood tests and imaging, including cholangiography
- TNM and Nevin's staging systems are used
- Surgery is the mainstay of treatment
- Radiotherapy or chemotherapy are only occasionally used
- Prognosis is poor

GASTRINOMA

- Gastrinomas are very rare and mainly occur in the duodenum or pancreas
- They are a neuroendocrine tumour and may be related to multiple endocrine neoplasia (MEN) type I or Zollinger-Ellison syndrome
- Symptoms are similar to peptic ulcer disease
- Fasting serum gastrin is a useful test
- Primary treatment is surgery, although chemotherapy can be used in non-resectable metastatic disease
- Proton pump inhibitors improve symptoms
- The presence of liver metastases has a significant impact upon prognosis

KEY POINTS SUMMARY

Oesophageal carcinoma

- Oesophageal carcinoma is the eighth most common malignancy in the UK
- Tumours occurring in the upper two thirds are usually squamous cell carcinoma, whilst those in the lower third are usually adenocarcinoma
- Smoking, alcohol consumption and obesity are important risk factors in western countries, but dietary factors play a significant role in the higher incidences areas such as Iran and China
- Dysphagia and weight loss are the most common presenting features, although lower third adenocarcinomas may be asymptomatic
- Surgery is the only realistic chance for cure, but is only possible in around a third of the patients that present
- Overall five year survival is 10-15%

Gastric carcinoma

- Gastric cancer is the sixth most common malignancy in the UK (and the fourth most common worldwide)
- It is the second most common cause of cancer death worldwide
- Helicobacter Pylori infection has a major aetiological role
- 95% of tumours are adenocarcinomas and half of all tumours occur in the pyloric region and a further quarter occur on the lesser curve
- Surgery is the only treatment modality that offers the potential of cure
- Surgery can also be used in the palliative setting
- Overall five year survival is 20%

Hepatocellular carcinoma

- Hepatocellular carcinoma is the sixth most common tumour worldwide, but is rare in the UK
- It tends to occur from regenerating nodules in a cirrhotic liver, and so the key risk factors are those that cause liver cirrhosis
- Patients often have no additional symptoms other than those that pre-exist with their chronic liver disease
- Even though the tumour does not commonly cause distant metastases, surgical resection is only possible in 10-15% of patients due to the size of the tumour coupled with the underlying poor liver function
- Overall five year survival is 3%

Pancreatic carcinoma

- Pancreatic cancer is the fifth most common cause of cancer death in the UK
- The main risk factors are smoking, obesity, low levels of exercise and chronic pancreatitis
- Presenting features are often vague, but most commonly include jaundice and weight loss
- 80% of pancreatic tumours are ductal adenocarcinomas
- 75% of tumours occur in the head of the pancreas
- Ca19.9 is not sensitive or specific enough as a diagnostic test, but has a role in assessing the effects of treatment and in follow up surveillance
- Surgery is the only treatment that offers a potential cure, but just 15% of patients have resectable disease at diagnosis
- Overall five year survival is 4%

Others

- The most common presenting features of anal cancer are rectal bleeding or discomfort. Most are squamous cell carcinomas and chemoradiation is the primary treatment modality
- Small bowel carcinoma most commonly affects the duodenum and proximal jejunum. The primary treatment is surgery
- Cholangiocarcinoma and tumours of the gallbladder have a poor prognosis
- Gastrinomas are very rare. It is important to look for the presence of liver metastases as this has a significant impact upon prognosis

LUNG CANCER

EPIDEMIOLOGY

- Lung cancer is the most common UK cancer
- In the UK, more patients die from lung cancer than breast and colorectal cancer combined
- It is more common in males than females

RISK FACTORS INCLUDE

- Smoking
- Exposure to passive smoking
- COPD
- Other pre-existing lung diseases
- Occupational exposures such as industrial dust
- Previous cancer, particularly of the head and neck

SCREENING/TYPES/ PATHOLOGY

- Lung cancer is broadly classified as small cell (SCLC) or non-small cell (NSCLC)
- SCLC makes up 20% of cases and metastasises early (85% beyond the thorax at diagnosis)
- SCLCs tend to contain membrane bound neurosecretory granules that can release calcitonin, ADH, ACTH and PTH related peptide
- NSCLC makes up the remaining 80% of cases and can be further classified as below
- Squamous cell carcinoma (45% of NSCLC) affects proximal, large bronchi and therefore can present with obstructive lesions (recurrent pneumonias are common). Local spread is common, but distant metastases occur late. They can also secrete PTH related peptide
- Adenocarcinoma (35% of NSCLC) is slow growing and tends to arise in scars in peripheral lung tissue. It is more common in women and is less strongly associated with smoking than other types.   It frequently metastasises to brain and bone
- Large cell carcinoma (10% of NSCLC) is less differentiated and tends to metastasise earlier than adenocarcinoma and squamous cell carcinoma
- Mixed histological types
- Carcinoid tumours
- Sarcoma
- Metastatic spread can be via local invasion, lymphatic spread or haematogenous routes
- There is no national screening programme for lung cancer in the UK

SIGNS & SYMPTOMS

- Cough +/- haemoptysis
- Dyspnoea
- Chest pain
- Recurrent pneumonia
- Hoarseness of voice
- Weight loss
- Fatigue
- Finger clubbing
- Supraclavicular or axillary lymphadenopathy
- Wheeze or stridor
- Pleural effusion
- Unexplained hyponatraemia
- Signs and symptoms of metastatic or paraneoplastic disease such as bone pain, hepatomegaly, confusion and proximal myopathy
- Pancoast/Horner syndromes
- Signs and symptoms of superior vena cava obstruction

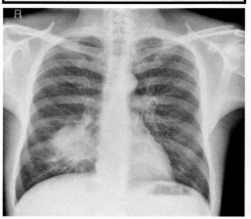

A large spiculated mass in the right lower lobe which is the typical appearance of a tumour

INVESTIGATIONS

- Blood tests
- Chest x-ray
- Sputum cytology
- Bronchoscopy with biopsy
- Pleural effusion cytology
- FNAC of enlarged lymph nodes
- CT of thorax and for staging
- Bone/PET scan
- Pulmonary function tests if surgery or radical radiotherapy is being considered

LUNG CANCER

TREATMENT OPTIONS

NSCLC

- Surgery with mediastinal lymph node sampling offers the best chance of cure as it is not particularly chemotherapy sensitive
- However, less than 50% have resectable disease at presentation
- Radiotherapy is offered if surgery is not appropriate
- Radiotherapy can be a radical treatment for some
- Chemotherapy can be offered in stage 3 or 4 disease, but has a limited role
- Tyrosine kinase inhibitors gefitinib and erlotinib can be used as a first line treatment in those that test receptor positive
- The response rate to tyrosine kinase inhibitors is better in females, non-smokers and those with adenocarcinoma
- Percutaneous radiofrequency ablation can be offered as a concurrent treatment and can be performed on more than one occasion
- Photodynamic therapy may be an option in early disease in those not fit for surgery

SCLC

- Surgery is not usually possible (as SCLC metastasises early)
- But it is much more chemotherapy sensitive than NSCLC (80% response rate, with complete response in 60%)
- Multidrug regimes are used
- Radiotherapy may be offered if there is a good response from initial chemotherapy

General

- Multidisciplinary team discussion
- Smoking cessation advice and assistance
- Radiotherapy can be very useful as a palliative treatment such as for bronchial obstruction, distressing haemoptysis, cough, chest pain, superior vena cava obstruction, bone and brain metastases and spinal cord compression
- Debulking surgery can be considered in bronchial obstruction or for distressing haemoptysis
- Stents can be an option for bronchial obstruction and in superior vena cava obstruction
- Opiates can help with dyspnoea and cough in addition to pain
- Bisphosphonates should be considered for bony metastases
- Aspiration or drainage +/- pleurodesis can provide relief from symptoms of pleural effusions

STAGING AND PROGNOSIS

- The TNM staging system is used
- The majority of those with SCLC, even if they respond to chemotherapy, will relapse, particularly within the first year
- The overall two year survival for SCLC is only 10%
- Five year survival for resectable NSCLC ranges from 55% for stage 1 disease to 18% for stage 3 disease
- Five year survival is 10% for non-resectable NSCLC

PLEURAL MESOTHELIOMA

- Mesothelioma is a malignancy of the pleura
- It can also affect other mesothelial linings, particularly in the abdomen
- Mesothelioma is much more common in males than females
- Age at diagnosis is most frequently between 50 and 75
- There is a very strong association with exposure to asbestos, but there is a long lag period between exposure and disease (at least 20 years in the majority of cases)
- Previous radiotherapy as part of treatment for lymphoma or testicular germ cell cancer also increases the risk of mesothelioma
- Chest pain and breathlessness are the key presenting symptoms
- Possible signs include pleural effusion, chest wall mass and those relating to underlying asbestosis
- Chest x-ray, CT scan and pleural biopsy are the key investigations
- Imaging usually shows pleural thickening and effusion
- Mesotheliomas can be classified into three major subtypes: epithelioid, sarcomatoid and biphasic (mixed)
- The TNM staging system is used
- Management options are extremely limited
- Surgery may be possible only in stage 1 disease
- Chemotherapy or radiotherapy do not seem to significantly improve survival but may still be offered to patients who have unresectable disease
- However, radiotherapy is often used prophylactically following biopsy or chest drain to reduce the risk of seeding
- Prognosis is poor with median survival being 8-12 months

KEY POINTS SUMMARY

Lung cancer
- Lung cancer is the most common cancer and the leading cause of cancer death in the UK
- Smoking is by far the most significant risk factor in the development of lung malignancy
- Lung cancer can be broadly classified into non-small cell and small cell types, and this is important as the extent of disease and treatment differs significantly
- Because small cell lung cancer tends to metastasise early, chemotherapy is an important treatment modality
- With non-small cell lung cancer, surgical resection offers the best chance of cure and chemotherapy has only a limited role
- Radiotherapy can have a significant role in symptom palliation
- Overall five year survival for all types of lung cancer is 9%

Mesothelioma
- Mesothelioma is strongly associated with previous exposure to asbestos, often as long as twenty years before diagnosis
- Treatment options are limited and prognosis is poor
- Overall five year survival is 8%

CANCER OF THE ORAL CAVITY

EPIDEMIOLOGY

- Oral cancer makes up 2% of malignant tumours diagnosed in the UK
- It is more common in men
- Peak age at diagnosis is between 40 and 70
- A higher incidence is seen in India and France

RISK FACTORS INCLUDE

- Smoking
- Chewing tobacco
- Excessive alcohol consumption
- Poor dental hygiene
- Betel quid chewing
- Human papilloma virus
- Immunosuppression
- Leukoplakia or erythroplakia

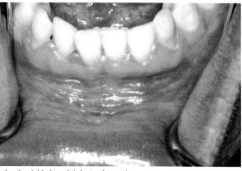

Leukoplakia is a risk factor for oral cancer

SIGNS & SYMPTOMS

- A non healing ulcer
- Persistent pain or discomfort
- Pain referred to the ear
- Speech difficulties
- Dysphagia
- Neck mass
- Local lymphadenopathy
- Weight loss

TYPES/PATHOLOGY/ SCREENING

- The oral cavity includes the lips, buccal mucosa, floor of the mouth, anterior two-thirds of the tongue, hard palate, gingiva and retromolar triangle
- The tongue is the most common site (35%)
- Over 90% are squamous cell carcinomas
- Other types include adenocarcinoma, adenoid cystic carcinoma, melanoma and lymphoma

INVESTIGATIONS

- Routine blood tests
- Orthopantomogram and chest x-ray
- Biopsy
- Nasoendoscopy
- FNAC of enlarged nodes
- CT or MRI scan

TREATMENT OPTIONS

- Referral to a dentist prior to treatment
- Multidisciplinary team discussion
- Early disease can be treated with either surgery or radiotherapy (external beam or brachytherapy)
- In advanced disease in fit individuals, the primary treatment is a radical resection with reconstruction
- Post operative radiotherapy may be considered
- Chemotherapy is considered in those with a high risk of recurrence (regimes usually include cisplatin or methotrexate)
- In those not fit for surgery, the best option is radical radiotherapy with concurrent chemotherapy
- Monoclonal antibody cetuximab may be considered

STAGING AND PROGNOSIS

- The TNM staging system is used
- Prognosis varies significantly by location, type and stage
- For tongue and oral cavity tumours (excluding lip) the overall five year survival is 56%

OTHER INTERESTING POINTS

- It is important to consider the effects of treatment; surgery can result in functional impairment, whereas radiotherapy often results in mucositis and xerostomia and may cause osteoradionecrosis
- A third of patients with tongue tumours develop further primary tumours

SALIVARY GLAND TUMOURS

EPIDEMIOLOGY

- Salivary gland tumours are rare, making up just 6% of head and neck tumours
- Most malignant tumours occur in those aged over 60
- There is an equal sex distribution of malignant tumours, but benign tumours are more common in women

RISK FACTORS INCLUDE

- Radiation exposure
- Smoking (but is mostly associated with Warthin's tumours)
- Previous skin cancer
- Viral infections, particularly HIV, Epstein Barr virus and human papilloma virus

SIGNS & SYMPTOMS

- Typically a slowly enlarging, painless mass
- The mass can sometimes cause pain
- Ulceration (particularly seen with minor glands within the oral cavity)
- Lymphadenopathy
- Facial nerve palsy
- Trismus
- Nasal congestion or obstruction
- Sinusitis
- Visual changes
- Dysphagia
- Sensory loss over the anterior two-thirds of the tongue
- Trigeminal nerve distribution pain

INVESTIGATIONS

- Ultrasound scan
- Followed by CT and/or MRI
- Ultrasound guided core biopsy or FNAC
- Routine blood tests
- Staging CT or PET scan

STAGING AND PROGNOSIS

- The TNM staging system is used
- Malignant parotid tumours tend to present late and therefore have a poor prognosis
- Minor salivary gland tumours have a better prognosis

TYPES/PATHOLOGY/ SCREENING

- The parotid gland is the commonest site (80% of tumours)
- However, tumours occurring in the other salivary glands are more likely to be malignant
- The most common benign tumour is a pleomorphic adenoma
- Other benign tumours include Warthin's tumour, basal cell adenoma and canalicular adenoma
- The most common malignant types are mucoepidermoid carcinoma and adenoid cystic carcinoma
- Adenocarcinoma, squamous cell carcinoma acinic cell carcinoma and mixed types also occur
- Metastatic spread is primarily to the lungs, but also to bone and to the liver
- Adenoid cystic carcinoma has a high risk of metastatic disease that can occur up to 20 years after initial diagnosis
- A rare but important type is the small cell carcinoma, (which occurs in less than 2% of cases, particularly in older men), due to it commonly having metastasised at diagnosis

TREATMENT OPTIONS

- Referral to a dentist prior to treatment
- Multidisciplinary team discussion
- Primary treatment is surgery
- The facial nerve is spared if possible
- Adjuvant radiotherapy can reduce the risk of recurrence
- Chemotherapy is only usually considered in advanced or recurrent disease

OTHER INTERESTING POINTS

- Tumours that result in facial nerve involvement are almost always malignant
- Other features that suggest a malignant lesion are hardness, fixation, tenderness and overlying ulceration
- Pain can occur with both malignant and benign tumours
- Frey's syndrome (erythema and sweating of the cheek) can occur on eating or even thinking about certain foods post parotid surgery

LARYNGEAL CANCER

EPIDEMIOLOGY

- Laryngeal cancer accounts for 1-2% of all malignancies in the UK, and is the second most common cancer of the head and neck
- Males are five times more commonly affected than females
- The peak age of onset is 50-70 years

RISK FACTORS INCLUDE

- Smoking
- Excessive alcohol
- Human papilloma virus
- Poor dental health
- Poor diet
- Family history of head and neck cancer
- Immunosuppression
- Some occupational exposures

SIGNS & SYMPTOMS

- Hoarseness or a change in voice
- Dysphagia
- Weight loss
- Cough
- Haemoptysis
- Dyspnoea
- Halitosis
- The sensation of a lump in the throat
- Fatigue
- Earache
- Lymphadenopathy

TYPES/PATHOLOGY/SCREENING

- Virtually all tumours are squamous cell carcinomas
- Adenocarcinoma, sarcoma, lymphoma or plasmacytoma can rarely occur
- Laryngeal cancers can be classified into the following types:
  - Glottic (60%), the most common and tends to present early
  - Supraglottic (30%) usually presents with more locally advanced disease
  - Subglottic (5%)
  - Marginal (5%)
- Lymphatic spread is to the deep cervical lymph nodes

INVESTIGATIONS

- Chest x-ray
- Flexible laryngoscopy
- Examination under anaesthetic with biopsy
- FNAC of enlarged lymph nodes
- Routine blood tests
- Ultrasound, CT, MRI and PET scans may be considered appropriate depending upon the presentation

TREATMENT OPTIONS

- Multidisciplinary team discussion
- For small, early tumours there are comparable results with both radiotherapy and surgery
- Radiotherapy is usually given five days a week, for several weeks
- Endoscopic surgery is often possible for small tumours
- For larger tumours a partial or total laryngectomy can be performed
- A block dissection may be needed if there is nodal disease
- Post-operative radiotherapy is usually offered in advanced disease
- Chemotherapy (usually platinum based), may be offered in advanced or recurrent disease and can be used neo-adjuvantly in some circumstances
- Monoclonal antibody cetuximab may be considered
- Post treatment input from a dietician and speech and language therapist is important

STAGING AND PROGNOSIS

- The TNM staging system is used
- Overall there is a 65% five year survival
- But in early disease this approaches 90%
- Glottic tumours have the best prognosis due to the earlier diagnosis because of the hoarseness of voice

OTHER INTERESTING POINTS

- The loss of voice following a total laryngectomy can cause great distress
- The three main ways to regain speech are tracheoesophageal puncture, oesophageal speech (swallowing air) or using an electrolarynx

RETINOBLASTOMA

EPIDEMIOLOGY

- Retinoblastoma is the most common eye malignancy of childhood
- There are around 50 cases a year in the UK and the incidence is increasing
- It mostly (97%) affects those aged under 5
- There is no sex or ethnicity predisposition
- A quarter of cases are bilateral
- Unilateral retinoblastoma is most common during the first two years of life, whereas bilateral cases most often occur between 24 and 36 months

RISK FACTORS INCLUDE

- Most unilateral cases are sporadic
- Bilateral disease is inherited
- It is the inheritance of an altered copy of the retinoblastoma gene (RB1 gene) that predisposes to retinoblastoma

SIGNS & SYMPTOMS

- The most common feature is leukocoria ('white eye')
- Strabismus
- Decreased vision
- Ocular inflammation
- Absence of the red reflex
- Iris heterochromia

TYPES/PATHOLOGY/ SCREENING

- This is a malignancy of early life as the retinal cells develop rapidly in the first few years and are usually fully developed by the age of 5
- The RB1 gene maps to chromosome 13 and encodes a tumour suppressor
- A 'two hit hypothesis' has been proposed to explain inherited forms, which is that one altered copy is inherited and the second becomes mutated in a retinal cell
- Untreated, retinoblastoma will grow to fill the eye and destroy the globe

INVESTIGATIONS

- Ophthalmoscopic examination
- CT/MRI
- Bone scan (see brown box)

TREATMENT OPTIONS

- Referral to a specialist centre; in the UK these are the Birmingham Children's Hospital and the Royal London Hospital
- Specific treatment depends upon the size and location of the tumour, visual prognosis, presence of seeds and the child's age
- Cryotherapy and/or laser photocoagulation or thermotherapy is an option for small tumours
- Combination chemotherapy is used for medium or large tumours
- This is usually as a chemoreduction technique to then allow other treatments but is also used for metastatic disease
- Surgery may involve enucleation (removal of the globe), particularly if there is little response to the above more conservative approaches
- Radiotherapy is effective, but is now less frequently used due to the risk of inducing future secondary malignancies
- Genetic counselling is also an important element of the management

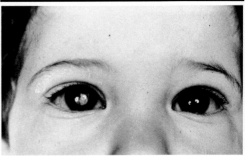

A child with retinoblastoma. Leukocoria can be discovered with home digital photography

STAGING AND PROGNOSIS

- The International Classification for Intraocular Retinoblastoma (ICIRB) is used for staging
- Overall five year survival is 94%
- However, the prognosis is very poor for metastatic disease

OTHER INTERESTING POINTS

- Those with an RB1 mutation are also at greater risk of developing a second primary malignancy, particularly sarcomas and melanoma

THYROID CANCER

EPIDEMIOLOGY

- Thyroid cancer is rare; it accounts for less than 1% of all malignancies diagnosed in the UK
- It is however the most common malignancy of the endocrine system
- Females are affected more than males

RISK FACTORS INCLUDE

- Benign thyroid disease, which includes adenomas, goitres and thyroiditis
- Family history of thyroid cancer
- Previous radiotherapy
- Exposure to other forms of radiation
- Familial adenomatous polyposis
- Acromegaly
- Previous benign breast lumps
- Being overweight or particularly tall

TYPES/PATHOLOGY/ SCREENING

- Papillary carcinomas are the most common thyroid tumours (65%) and tend to occur in younger patients and are slow growing therefore giving a good prognosis
- Follicular tumours make up around 15% of thyroid cancers, and tend to occur in middle age patients, particularly those who are iodine deficient
- Follicular carcinoma has a greater propensity than papillary carcinoma to metastasise, particularly to the lungs and bone
- Hürthle cell carcinoma is a cytological variant of follicular carcinoma and tends to behave more aggressively
- Medullary carcinoma accounts for around 6% of cases, and whilst most (75%) are sporadic, some are familial as part of the multiple neoplasia type 2 (MEN2) syndrome
- Medullary carcinomas are more aggressive than the more well differentiated papillary and follicular carcinomas
- Anaplastic carcinoma makes up around 7% of cases, tends to occur in those aged over 60 and carries a poor prognosis
- At least half of patients with anaplastic carcinoma present with metastatic disease affecting the lungs, bone, liver and/or brain
- Non-Hodgkin's lymphoma, makes up about 1% of cases, and classically occurs in women aged over 50 with Hashimoto's thyroiditis

SIGNS & SYMPTOMS

- Neck swelling
- A discrete thyroid nodule
- A persistent sore throat
- Symptoms of compression in advanced disease such as a hoarse voice, dysphagia or stridor
- Most patients are euthyroid
- Medullary thyroid cancer can cause additional symptoms related to calcitonin such as facial flushing and loose stools

INVESTIGATIONS

- Thyroid function tests and thyroid antibodies
- Ultrasound scan
- FNAC
- CT staging scan
- Thyroid isotope scan
- PET scan

TREATMENT OPTIONS

- Multidisciplinary team discussion
- Surgical resection is the primary treatment
- However, most anaplastic carcinomas are not resectable due to local spread at diagnosis
- A selective lymph node resection is also usually performed
- Following surgery for papillary or follicular tumours remaining thyroid tissue may be ablated with radioactive iodine (iodine-131)
- As medullary and anaplastic carcinomas don't pick up iodine very well, external beam radiotherapy is preferred
- Hormonal treatment with thyroxine to suppress TSH secretion can slow the growth of tumours and reduce the risk of recurrence
- The role of chemotherapy tends to be in advanced disease or recurrence
- Other options include tyrosine kinase inhibitors; vandetanib for medullary carcinoma or sorafenib for papillary and follicular carcinomas

STAGING AND PROGNOSIS

- The TNM staging system is used
- On the whole prognosis is good with a five year survival of 86%, however for anaplastic carcinoma for which there is no effective treatment, five year survival is less than 5%

OTHERS

CARCINOMA OF THE LIP

- Carcinoma of the lip makes up around 25% of oral malignancies
- It is more common in males and Caucasians
- Risk factors include sun damage, smoking (especially pipe smoking) and leukoplakia
- It affects the lower lip in 95% of cases
- Most tumours are squamous cell carcinomas
- It most commonly metastasises to the submandibular nodes, although less than 10% of patients present with nodal spread
- Investigations include biopsy of the lesion and FNAC of any enlarged lymph nodes
- No further investigations are usually needed unless there is clinical evidence of advance disease
- The TNM staging system is used
- Surgery and radiotherapy give comparable results
- Cure rate is around 90%

NASOPHARYNGEAL CARCINOMA

- Nasopharyngeal carcinoma is rare in the UK (around 250 cases a year) but is endemic in Southern China
- Males are at increased risk and the peak age of onset is between 50 and 60 years of age
- Risk factors include poor diet, smoking, Epstein-Barr virus, family history and chronic ear, nose and throat conditions
- Presenting features include hearing loss and/or tinnitus, headache, lymphadenopathy and nasal obstruction
- The WHO has classified nasopharyngeal carcinoma by histological type; these are keratinising squamous cell carcinoma (type I), differentiated nonkeratinising carcinoma (type II), undifferentiated nonkeratinising carcinoma (type III) and basaloid squamous cell carcinoma
- Adenocarcinoma, adenoid cystic carcinoma, lymphoma, melanoma and sarcoma can rarely occur
- Investigations include nasoendoscopy and/or panendoscopy, biopsy, FNAC of enlarged lymph nodes and CT, MRI and/or PET scans
- The primary treatment is radiotherapy
- Due to the anatomical location, surgery is seldom possible but concurrent chemotherapy may be used, particularly in younger patients
- The TNM staging system is used
- Overall five year survival is 50%

PARATHYROID CARCINOMA

- Parathyroid carcinoma is a very rare tumour, making up just 1-2% of cases of primary hyperparathyroidism
- Even though hyperparathyroidism is more common in females, parathyroid carcinoma has no sex predisposition
- Mutation of the HRPT2 tumour suppressor gene is thought to play a significant role in the pathogenesis
- The most common presenting complaint is symptomatic hypercalcaemia, and particularly bone and renal symptoms
- Just under half of patients will have a neck mass and up to 15% can present with pancreatitis
- Due to non-specific features, histological diagnosis is difficult
- Surgery is the mainstay of definitive treatment, but many patients will require treatment of their hypercalcaemia first
- Studies looking at adjuvant chemotherapy or radiotherapy have yielded poor results
- About one third of patients experience an aggressive disease course, a third are cured by initial or follow up surgery and a third have a relapse of disease
- Overall five year survival is around 50%

PARANASAL SINUS TUMOURS

- Paranasal sinus tumours (maxillary, ethmoid, frontal and sphenoid) are well differentiated squamous cell carcinomas in more than 50% of cases
- Most of the remaining tumours are adenocarcinomas, adenoid cystic carcinomas and mucoepidermoid carcinomas
- Human papilloma virus, smoking and exposure to certain chemicals (particularly wood dust, leather dust, chromium, nickel, formaldehyde and cloth fibres) are the key risk factors
- They tend to present late as they don't tend to initially cause any symptoms
- The most common features are swelling, nasal congestion and pain, but there may also be ocular symptoms or dental symptoms depending upon location and extension
- Treatment is surgery with reconstruction, followed usually by adjuvant radiotherapy
- The additional use of chemotherapy is growing in popularity in an attempt to further reduce the risk of recurrence

KEY POINTS SUMMARY

Overall
- Head and neck cancers are responsible for 3% of cancer deaths in the UK
- Most share smoking and excessive alcohol consumption as key aetiological factors
- Most tumours are squamous cell carcinomas
- Patients with early disease are often treated with a single modality, usually surgery or radiotherapy, but in more advanced disease a multimodality treatment approach is preferred
- Treatment of the cervical lymph nodes is frequently performed, even when disease here is not clinically detected due to the frequency of occult metastases to these nodes

Cancer of the oral cavity
- Oral cancer makes up 2% of malignancies diagnosed in the UK
- Smoking, excessive alcohol consumption and poor dental hygiene are the key risk factors
- The tongue is the most common site and the vast majority are squamous cell carcinomas
- Early disease can be treated with either surgery or radiotherapy, but in more advanced disease surgery with adjuvant radiotherapy and/or chemotherapy is the best option
- Overall five year survival is 56%

Cancer of the salivary glands
- Salivary gland tumours make up just 6% of tumours of the head and neck
- Most patients present with a slow growing swelling or mass
- Whilst most tumours occur in the parotid gland, it is tumours in the other glands that are more likely to be malignant
- Hardness, fixation, tenderness, overlying ulceration and involvement of the facial nerve are suggestive of a malignant lesion
- The primary treatment is surgery
- Overall five year survival is 69%

Laryngeal cancer
- Laryngeal cancer is the second most common head and neck malignancy
- Glottic tumours are the most common and have a good prognosis as they tend to present early with hoarseness of voice
- For early disease the results from treatment with surgery or radiotherapy are comparable, but for larger tumours, surgery is preferred where possible
- The three main ways to regain speech after laryngectomy are tracheoesophageal puncture, oesophageal speech (swallowing air) or using an electrolarynx
- Overall five year survival is 65%

Retinoblastoma
- There are around 50 cases of retinoblastoma diagnosed in the UK each year
- Leukocoria is the most common presenting feature
- Bilateral cases are inherited, whilst unilateral cases are more likely to be sporadic
- Overall five year survival is 94%

Thyroid cancer
- Thyroid cancer accounts for less than 1% of all cancers diagnosed in the UK
- Papillary and follicular carcinomas are the most common forms
- Patients tend to be euthyroid
- Surgery is the primary treatment
- Overall five year survival is 86%

Others
- Due to the anatomical location, surgery is seldom possible for nasopharyngeal carcinoma
- Parathyroid carcinoma makes up just 1-2% of cases of primary hyperparathyroidism

BREAST CANCER

EPIDEMIOLOGY

- The life time risk of breast cancer is 1 in 9 for females, representing 1 in 3 malignancies in females
- It is the leading cause of death amongst females aged 35-55 in western countries
- However, incidence increases with age and 75% of cases occur in those aged over 50
- Around 0.5% of cases occur in males
- The incidence of breast cancer is increasing in developed countries, but the death rate is falling (probably due to screening and improved treatment)
- Interestingly, breast cancer is more frequently diagnosed in women of a higher social economic status (although lower social economic classes have a worse prognosis)

RISK FACTORS INCLUDE

- Family history (particularly sister or mother and of early onset)
- Other genetic factors (the BRCA1, BRCA2 and TP53 genes predispose, but they only represent 5% of breast cancers)
- Prolonged oestrogen exposure (early menarche, late menopause, nulliparity, late first pregnancy and obesity, particularly post menopausal obesity)
- Lifestyle (particularly obesity, alcohol intake and saturated fats)
- Hormone replacement therapy and oral contraceptives (conveys a slightly increased risk that declines after use)
- Hormone replacement therapy can increase the risk by 35% after five years of use
- Previous irradiation to the chest

SIGNS & SYMPTOMS

- May be asymptomatic (found by screening in around 15-20%)
- Breast lump (85%)
- Breast pain (5%; breast cancer usually presents with a painless lump)
- Nipple changes such as retraction, discharge, or rash as in Paget's disease
- Skin changes such as dimpling or tethering
- Lymphadenopathy, particularly in the axilla
- Symptoms associated with metastatic disease such as bone pain
- Sometimes, usually elderly patients, present with a fungating tumour that has been neglected

SCREENING/TYPES/ PATHOLOGY

- Classification of types includes
- Ductal carcinoma in situ (DCIS, is preinvasive as it does not breach the basement membrane)
- Lobular carcinoma in situ (has a 25% 20 year risk of developing invasive carcinoma)
- Ductal carcinoma (by far the most common invasive tumour making up 80% of tumours)
- Infiltrating lobular carcinoma (around 10% of tumours, but they have an increased incidence of being bilateral tumours)
- Colloid (mucinous) carcinoma (makes up less than 5% of tumours, but has a good prognosis)
- Other types which have a reasonable prognosis include medullary carcinoma, tubular carcinoma, cribriform carcinoma and papillary carcinoma
- Paget's disease of the breast, squamous cell carcinoma and inflammatory carcinoma are other types, but the prognosis is not so good
- In addition to the type the pathologist will also report the receptor status as this will have implications for the types of treatment that can be offered
- The receptor reporting typically includes oestrogen receptor status, progesterone receptor status and Human Epidermal Growth Factor Receptor 2 (HER2) status
- Breast cancer commonly metastasises to lung, bone, liver and brain
- In the UK all women aged 50-70 are invited for three yearly screening, which involves a clinical examination and mammography
- Those attending for screening have a breast cancer mortality risk reduction of between 15% and 40%
- 5mm tumours can be detected by a mammogram
- Mammography in women aged under 50 has not demonstrated a significant improvement in mortality (likely due to denser breast tissue) and MRI (or ultrasound) is a better option in high risk young women
- Tests such as the CA15.3 tumour marker can be useful for prognosis, but does not have a role in screening or diagnosis
- Genetic testing is considered when there is a significant likelihood of finding a gene mutation
- Genetic counselling is important if genetic testing is being considered due to the additional implications

BREAST CANCER

INVESTIGATIONS

- The key to assessment and diagnosis is the 'triple assessment' involving clinical examination, imaging and biopsy
- Ultrasound is sometimes preferred to mammograms in 'one stop clinics' especially in younger patients
- MRI has a particular role in the young (under 50), those with breast implants and those that have had previous surgery or radiotherapy
- Biopsy may be FNAC, core or vacuum assisted
- Blood tests including LFTs
- Staging CT scan
- PET scan

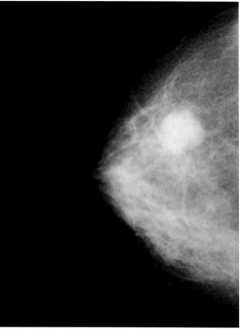

An abnormal mammogram

TREATMENT OPTIONS

- Multidisciplinary team discussion
- Surgery is the mainstay of treatment
- The two broad types of surgery are breast conserving or mastectomy (with or without reconstruction)
- Survival rates for breast conserving surgery (when appropriate) and mastectomy are comparable as long as the appropriate adjuvant therapy is given
- Axillary biopsy/sampling +/- clearance is important for prognosis
- The Nottingham prognostic index may be calculated to help assess benefit of adjuvant treatments
- Whole breast radiotherapy is recommended after all breast conserving surgery and in mastectomy patients with either large tumours or at least four positive axillary nodes
- Adjuvant hormonal therapy, such as tamoxifen or anastrozole can be used if the tumour is receptor positive
- Adjuvant chemotherapy is important in hormone receptor negative patients due to the risk of occult micrometastasis (which can present many years later)
- Chemotherapy agents that are frequently used include anthracyclines, paclitaxel, docetaxel, vinorelbine and capecitabine
- In HER2 positive disease, monoclonal antibody trastuzumab (Herceptin) is effective
- Supportive care that also takes into account the psychological aspects of breast cancer is important
- Radiotherapy can have a further role in metastatic disease to the brain or bone
- Bisphosphonates are indicated for multiple bony metastases

STAGING AND PROGNOSIS

- The TNM staging system is used
- Axillary node status is the best indicator of prognosis
- The Nottingham prognostic index can also be used
- Overall prognosis varies widely, and five year survival ranges from 95% for DCIS to 15% for stage 4 disease

MALE BREAST CANCER

- 1 in 200 cases of breast cancer are diagnosed in males
- Over 90% are oestrogen and/or progesterone receptor positive
- Risk factors include family history, increased exposure to oestrogens, lifestyle factors and increasing age
- Prognosis is similar to that of female breast cancer and the Nottingham prognostic index can be used
- However, there is often a delay in diagnosis (due to late presentation and more than 40% of patients have stage 3 or 4 disease at diagnosis) and so overall mortality is higher than in females

KEY POINTS SUMMARY

Breast cancer
- The life time risk of breast cancer for females is 1 in 9
- Although family history is an important risk factor only 5% of cases are due to inherited genes
- Prolonged oestrogen exposure is also a key risk factor
- A painless breast lump is the most frequent presenting feature, although around 15% of cases are in asymptomatic women which are discovered at screening
- Ductal carcinoma is the most common invasive tumour type
- Surgery is the mainstay of treatment
- The Nottingham prognostic index may be calculated to help assess benefit of adjuvant treatments
- Overall five year survival is 85%

Male breast cancer
- 0.5% of cases of breast cancer are diagnosed in males
- Over 90% are oestrogen and/or progesterone receptor positive
- Although prognosis is comparable to female breast cancer when comparing like for like disease stage, breast cancer in males tends to be diagnosed later and so the mortality rate is higher

RENAL CELL CARCINOMA

EPIDEMIOLOGY

- Renal cell carcinoma makes up 3% of all adult cancers
- The incidence is increasing
- It is more common in males
- The peak age of onset is between 40 and 70

RISK FACTORS INCLUDE

- Smoking
- Obesity
- Chronic kidney disease, particularly acquired renal cystic disease or any form leading to long term dialysis
- Genetic disorders such as Von Hippel-Lindau syndrome and tuberous sclerosis
- Hypertension
- Exposure to cadmium
- Thyroid cancer
- Radiotherapy

SIGNS & SYMPTOMS

- Classically, the triad of frank haematuria, loin pain and a loin mass
- Anaemia
- Constitutional symptoms such as fatigue, weight loss and night sweats
- Occasionally renal cell carcinoma can present as a paraneoplastic syndrome with pyrexia of unknown origin, polycythaemia, high output heart failure (arteriovenous shunts within the tumour), hypercalcaemia, or renin induced hypertension

TYPES/PATHOLOGY/ SCREENING

- Renal cell carcinoma makes up around 85% of neoplasms of the kidney
- Renal cell carcinoma is regarded as an adenocarcinoma of the proximal renal tubule
- Types include clear cell (85%), papillary (10%, which are more commonly bilateral and multifocal), chromophobe (4%) and collecting duct (Bellini's tumour, 1%)
- Other types of renal tumours include transitional cell carcinomas, sarcomatoid and oncocytomas
- Method of spread is haematogenous and the most common site is the lungs
- Bone, brain, liver and the other kidney are other frequent sites of metastatic disease

INVESTIGATIONS

- Urine dipstick, microscopy and culture
- Blood tests including U&Es and calcium
- Abdominal ultrasound
- CT urogram
- Intravenous pyelogram
- Cystoscopy (to exclude bladder cancer as a cause of haematuria)
- Renal angiogram/venogram and CT scanning for surgical planning (looking for renal vein or contralateral involvement)
- Chest x-ray
- CT/MRI for staging
- Bone scan if bony metastases suspected

TREATMENT OPTIONS

- Multidisciplinary team discussion
- Surgery is the mainstay of treatment, particularly in localised disease
- Surgery tends to involve partial or whole nephrectomy
- Percutaneous radiofrequency ablation, laparoscopic cryotherapy, percutaneous cryotherapy, irreversible electroporation and renal artery embolisation may be options in those not fit for nephrectomy
- Renal tumours do not tend to respond to chemotherapy even in metastatic disease
- Radiotherapy also tends to be ineffective but can have a role however in palliation of bony or brain metastases
- In metastatic or advanced disease, biological therapy such as with interleukin-2, interferon alpha or sunitinib may be appropriate
- Metastasectomy should be performed when possible

STAGING AND PROGNOSIS

- The TNM staging system is used
- Overall five year survival is 30-50%
- There is a significant association between older age at presentation and poorer prognosis

OTHER INTERESTING POINTS

- Von Hippel-Lindau syndrome is an autosomal dominant condition that as well as clear cell renal cancer, also predisposes to the development of haemangioblastomas, retinal angiomas and phaeochromocytomas

BLADDER CANCER

EPIDEMIOLOGY

- Bladder carcinoma is the fourth most common cancer in males (eleventh in females)
- It is more common in industrialised countries and in those aged over 65

RISK FACTORS INCLUDE

- Smoking
- Aniline dyes
- Polycyclic hydrocarbons
- Previous cyclophosphamide or radiotherapy
- BPH and associated surgery
- Recurrent UTIs, bladder calculi or other chronic irritation (particularly for squamous cell carcinoma)
- Type 2 diabetes mellitus

SIGNS & SYMPTOMS

- Painless haematuria (in 90%)
- Dysuria, urinary frequency, urgency or loin pain, particularly in advanced disease
- Signs and symptoms of metastatic disease

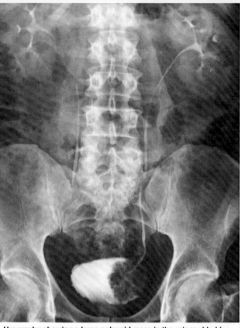

Urography showing a large polypoid mass in the urinary bladder

INVESTIGATIONS

- Urine dipstick, microscopy, culture and cytology
- Cystoscopy with biopsy
- Abdominal ultrasound
- Intravenous urogram
- CT/MRI scan for staging
- PET/bone scan

TYPES/PATHOLOGY/ SCREENING

- Transitional cell carcinoma is the most common form (85%)
- Transitional cell carcinoma can be divided into carcinoma in situ (10% at presentation), superficial (often papillary) growths (60%) and invasive (30%)
- Other types of tumour include squamous cell carcinoma (5%, although more common in developing countries, particularly due to schistosomiasis and other chronic irritation), adenocarcinoma (2%), sarcoma and lymphoma
- Only 5% of cases have metastasised at presentation, but common sites include lymph nodes, lungs and bone

TREATMENT OPTIONS

- Multidisciplinary team discussion

In superficial disease
- Transurethral resection of bladder tumours (TURBT)
- Adjuvant intravesical chemotherapy post surgery lowers the rate of recurrence; mitomycin, epirubicin and doxorubicin are frequently used agents
- Tuberculosis vaccination can be used as intravesical immunotherapy

Invasive disease
- Partial or radical cystectomy with urostomy formation
- Radiotherapy is a reasonable option in those not fit for surgery
- Systemic chemotherapy (often cisplatin based) can be used adjuvantly, neo-adjuvantly, with radiotherapy or palliatively

STAGING AND PROGNOSIS

- The TNM staging system is used
- Overall five year survival is 57% for males and 47% for females
- The recurrence rate for transitional cell carcinoma is high (70% within five years)

PROSTATE CANCER

EPIDEMIOLOGY

- Prostate cancer makes up 15-20% of all male cancers
- The incidence rate is 130 per 100,000 males and incidence increases with advancing age
- It is more common amongst North American and European men, particularly of Afro-Caribbean decent

RISK FACTORS INCLUDE

- Family history of prostate or breast cancer
- Western diet of high fat with low exercise
- Dietary selenium, vitamin E and lycopene (tomatoes) may be protective

SIGNS & SYMPTOMS

- Obstructive symptoms such as urgency, hesitancy, poor urinary flow, frequency (especially nocturnal) and haematuria
- Haematospermia
- Bone pain from metastases may be the presenting complaint
- Lymphadenopathy
- Hard craggy prostate on PR examination

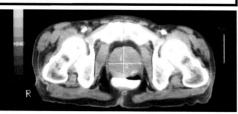

A CT scan showing a grossly enlarged prostate

TYPES/PATHOLOGY/ SCREENING

- 95% are adenocarcinoma and the remainder are transitional cell or neuroendocrine
- Most arise from the peripheral zone meaning symptoms present later than with benign prostatic hypertrophy which affects the central zones
- Prostate cancer is graded using a Gleason Score which reflects differentiation
- Poor differentiation is associated with disease spread
- Bone metastases are common, as is lymphatic spread to pelvic nodes
- Trials for screening in the UK with PSA levels did not improve outcomes

INVESTIGATIONS

- Blood tests including a PSA
- Urinalysis
- Rectal ultrasound with transrectal prostate biopsy
- Transperineal template biopsy
- Bone scan
- CT/MRI scan for staging

TREATMENT OPTIONS

- Multidisciplinary team discussion
- Watchful waiting may be appropriate for low grade, asymptomatic tumours in those that are poor surgical candidates
- Surgical options include a transurethral resection of prostate (not curative, but relieves symptoms and provides histology) or a radical prostatectomy (which can be curative)
- External beam radiotherapy or brachytherapy produces similar survival rates to surgery
- Radiotherapy also has a palliative role for bony metastases or prostatic bleeding
- Cryotherapy and high intensity focused ultrasound may be an option for recurrent or refractory disease
- Hormone therapy is the mainstay of treatment for metastatic disease as 80% of tumours are androgen deprivation responsive
- Chemotherapy can be used in hormone refractory prostate cancer
- It is also important to consider the wider management such as referral to erectile dysfunction services, bladder retraining and bisphosphonates in bone metastases

STAGING AND PROGNOSIS

- The TNM staging system is used
  - T1 microscopic
  - T2 macroscopic but within prostate gland
  - T3 invasion through the capsule
  - T4 invasion into other pelvic structures
- Prognosis varies widely upon grade and stage, but overall five year survival in the UK is 81%

OTHER INTERESTING POINTS

- The PSA level can be raised in other conditions such as benign prostatic hypertrophy, prostatitis, urinary retention and post urinary tract infection

TESTICULAR CANCER

EPIDEMIOLOGY

- Testicular cancer is the most common malignancy in men aged 20-40
- There are over 2000 new cases per year in the UK and the incidence is increasing

RISK FACTORS INCLUDE

- Cryptorchidism
- Family history of testicular cancer
- Previous testicular carcinoma in situ
- Infertility
- Hypospadias
- Inguinal hernia
- Immunosuppression (including HIV)
- Tall stature
- Klinefelter's syndrome

SIGNS & SYMPTOMS

- Most patients present with a painless unilateral testicular swelling
- One third have scrotal pain
- Lower abdominal discomfort
- Gynaecomastia
- Lymphadenopathy
- Constitutional symptoms such as fatigue and weight loss
- Signs and symptoms of metastatic spread such as backache, dyspnoea or dysphagia

TYPES/PATHOLOGY/SCREENING

- Most testicular cancers (95%) are germ cell tumours that can be split into:
  - Seminomas (40%) which can be further classified as classical, lymphocytic or syncytiotrophoblastic
  - Teratoma (40%) that can be further classified as differentiated, intermediate, undifferentiated or trophoblastic
  - Mixed seminoma/teratoma (15%)
- Other tumour types include yolk sac tumours, lymphoma, embryonal carcinoma, and choriocarcinoma
- Testicular tumours most commonly metastasise to the lungs, but also to the liver and brain
- There is no national screening programme, but the public are encouraged to actively self examine

INVESTIGATIONS

- Tumour markers including alpha-fetoprotein, human chorionic gonadotropin and lactate dehydrogenase
- Scrotal ultrasound
- Chest x-ray
- CT/MRI scan for staging
- Histology following orchidectomy

TREATMENT OPTIONS

- Multidisciplinary team discussion
- Counselling and sperm banking
- Orchidectomy, usually with insertion of a prosthesis
- Retroperitoneal or para-aortic lymph node dissection can be considered in cases of lymphatic spread
- Radiotherapy can be used to treat lymphatic spread of seminomas
- Chemotherapy can be used in cases of lymph node spread or distant metastasis
- Commonly used chemotherapy agents include carboplatin, bleomycin and etoposide

STAGING AND PROGNOSIS

- The TNM staging system can be used
- Alternatives include the Royal Marsden staging
  - In stage 1 the tumour is confined to the testicle
  - In stage 2 pelvic and abdominal lymph nodes are involved
  - In stage 3 there is supradiaphragmatic lymph node spread
  - In stage 4 there is extralymphatic spread (usually lung and liver involvement)
- Overall five year survival is 95%
- Even significant metastatic disease is potentially curable
- Teratomas have a significant relapse rate (20-25%), most within the first year following initial treatment, but they still have an excellent response to chemotherapy
- Choriocarcinomas have a poor prognosis

OTHER INTERESTING POINTS

- Biopsies of the testicle are not often performed due to the risk of seeding malignant cells with the biopsy needle

CERVICAL CANCER

EPIDEMIOLOGY

- Cervical cancer is the second most common female malignancy worldwide and accounts for around 2% of female malignancies in the UK
- There are two peaks of incidence; in the third decade for in situ disease and over 50 years of age for invasive disease

RISK FACTORS INCLUDE

- Human papilloma virus (HPV), particularly types 16 and 18
- Smoking (squamous cell carcinoma only)
- Multiple sexual partners
- Sexually transmitted infections
- Chronic cervicitis
- Immunosuppression
- Non attendance at screening

SIGNS & SYMPTOMS

- Vaginal bleeding; intermenstrual, post-coital and/or post menopausal
- Vaginal discharge
- Dyspareunia, vaginal discomfort, rectal and bladder symptoms tend to occur later
- Signs of metastatic disease such as pelvic lymphadenopathy, ascites or pleural effusions

TYPES/PATHOLOGY/ SCREENING

- Cervical cancers usually originate from the squamocolumnar junction
- Squamous cell carcinomas (85%) originate from the ectocervix
- Adenocarcinomas (15%) originate from the endocervix
- The national screening programme for women in England consists of three yearly smear tests between the ages of 25 and 49 and then five yearly until aged 64
- In Scotland and Wales there is three yearly smear testing until the ages of 60 and 65 respectively
- Brushings from the squamocolumnar junction are sent for cytology
- Screening may show mild, moderate or severe dyskaryosis, or may be classed as CIN:
- CIN 1 involves a third of the epithelium
- CIN 2 involves two thirds of the epithelium
- CIN 3 involves the full thickness of epithelium

INVESTIGATIONS

- Most early cervical cancers are detected by the screening programme
- Once cervical cancer has been confirmed, the following may be required:
- Examination under anaesthetic; bimanual and rectal examination, hysteroscopy +/- sigmoidoscopy or cystoscopy
- Transrectal ultrasound and IV urogram
- Chest x-ray and CT staging scan
- Pelvic MRI
- PET CT for distal spread

TREATMENT OPTIONS

- Multidisciplinary team discussion
- Colposcopy is performed following abnormal smear test results
- Localised treatments include laser ablation, cold coagulation and cryotherapy
- LLETZ (large loop excision of the transformation zone), cone biopsy and hysterectomy are the main options to remove the whole transformation zone following more high risk smear results
- Complex surgery can be performed in locally advanced cancers; total pelvic exenteration removes all the gynaecological organs as well as the rectum and bladder
- Radiotherapy can be used to cure early cancers or be given adjuvantly as either brachytherapy or external beam
- Chemotherapy can be used in reoccurrence or in combination with radiotherapy in advanced disease

STAGING AND PROGNOSIS

- The FIGO system of staging is used
  - Stage 0: Carcinoma in situ
  - Stage 1: Confined to the cervix
  - Stage 2: Spread beyond the cervix such as to the vaginal wall
  - Stage 3: Pelvic spread that may involve the pelvic wall or ureters
  - Stage 4: Metastatic disease
- Five year survival is 80-98% in stage 1 disease, but is 20% in stage 4 disease

OTHER INTERESTING POINTS

- A HPV vaccination programme was started in 2008 for 12-13 year old girls

ENDOMETRIAL CANCER

EPIDEMIOLOGY

- Endometrial cancer is the fourth most common cancer in women
- The incidence is 26 cases per 100,000
- It most commonly affects those that are post menopausal
- It is most common in western society, however worldwide incidence is on the increase

RISK FACTORS INCLUDE

- Endometrial hyperplasia
- Unopposed oestrogen exposure
- Early menarche and late menopause
- Increased BMI
- Nulliparity
- Family history
- Hormone replacement therapy and high oestrogen contraceptive pills
- Tamoxifen
- Diabetes mellitus
- Polycystic ovary syndrome
- Hereditary nonpolyposis colon cancer
- Smoking and the combined OCP may be protective

SIGNS & SYMPTOMS

- Vaginal bleeding, particularly post menopausal, but also intermenstrual in younger age groups
- Vaginal discharge
- Pelvic pain, dyspareunia, weight loss and constitutional symptoms are suggestive of advanced disease
- Clinical examination may be normal in non advanced disease
- A smear test may show clumps of adenocarcinoma

TYPES/PATHOLOGY/SCREENING

- 90% are adenocarcinomas which tend to be one of three main types: Endometrioid (the most common), papillary serous (the most aggressive form) or clear cell
- The remaining 10% are adeno-acanthomas, leiomyosarcomas or adenosarcomas
- Direct extension is the most common form of spread, but metastasises, particularly to the lungs, bones, liver and brain can occur

INVESTIGATIONS

- Pelvic examination
- CA125 can be elevated
- Transvaginal ultrasound
- Endometrial biopsy via pipille, hysteroscopy or dilation and curettage
- Chest x-ray and CT or MRI for staging in more advanced disease
- Examination under anaesthetic +/- cystoscopy and proctoscopy

TREATMENT OPTIONS

- Multidisciplinary team discussion
- Hysterectomy and bilateral oophorectomy is often curative
- Lymph node sampling +/- clearance
- Radiotherapy may be used radically in locally advanced tumours or in those not fit for surgery
- Radiotherapy can also be used adjuvantly in higher stages of endometrial cancer
- Either external beam radiotherapy or brachytherapy can be used
- Oral progesterone can be used to treat stage 3 and 4 disease
- This hormonal treatment has a low response rate, but is very well tolerated as it is non-toxic and tends to increase general well being
- Chemotherapy can be given in combination with radiotherapy in high risk disease or on its own in palliation

STAGING AND PROGNOSIS

- The FIGO staging system is used:
- Stage 1: Limited to the uterus but may invade the myometrium
- Stage 2: Involvement of the cervix
- Stage 3: Spread to ovaries, vagina or lymph nodes
- Stage 4: Distant metastases
- Overall five year survival is 80%

OTHER INTERESTING POINTS

- At diagnosis, 75% of tumours are confined to the uterus
- This is because they tend to present relatively early with menstrual abnormalities leading to a reasonable prognosis

OVARIAN CANCER

EPIDEMIOLOGY

- Ovarian cancer is the fifth most common female malignancy
- The incidence is 20 cases per 100,000
- It is most common in those aged over 50

RISK FACTORS INCLUDE

- Family history of breast, ovarian, endometrial or bowel cancer (BRCA1, but also the BRCA2 mutation is important)
- Nulliparity, infertility or late first pregnancy
- Hormone replacement therapy
- Endometriosis (clear cell carcinoma)
- Previous ovarian cysts
- Smoking and high fat diet
- Breast feeding and the oral contraceptive pill can be protective

SIGNS & SYMPTOMS

- It is often asymptomatic in the early stages
- Lower abdominal pain
- Bloating, distension or ascites
- Irregular menstruation
- Abnormal vaginal bleeding, particularly post-menopausal bleeding
- Weight loss and fatigue
- Abdominal mass
- Urinary or bowel symptoms
- Back pain
- Dyspareunia

TYPES/PATHOLOGY/ SCREENING

- There is no national screening programme, but high risk women who have a significant family history should be referred to a clinical genetics service
- 90% of ovarian cancers are epithelial and can be subclassified into:
  - Serous cystadenocarcinoma (commonest)
  - Mucinous cystadenocarcinoma
  - Endometrioid carcinoma
  - Undifferentiated
  - Clear cell carcinoma
- The remainder are rare tumours, such as germ cell teratomas and sarcomas
- Tumours are graded as being well, moderately or poorly differentiated

INVESTIGATIONS

- Abdominal and bimanual examination
- CA125 tumour marker (elevated in 80% of cases)
- Transvaginal and abdominal ultrasound
- Ultrasound guided biopsy
- Staging CT scan
- Laparoscopy
- Ascitic tap for cytology

TREATMENT OPTIONS

- Multidisciplinary team discussion
- Surgery is the mainstay of treatment
- Oophorectomy which may be unilateral or bilateral depending on stage
- In more advanced disease, hysterectomy, oophorectomy and omentectomy can be performed
- Biopsies of lymph nodes, diaphragm and peritoneum may be taken
- Chemotherapy can be used adjuvantly, neo-adjuvantly, palliatively or in recurrent disease
- Carboplatin +/- paclitaxel is the mainstay
- Radiotherapy is seldom used due to side effects

STAGING AND PROGNOSIS

- The FIGO staging system is used:
  - Stage 1: Limited to the ovaries or in the peritoneal fluid
  - Stage 2: Pelvic disease
  - Stage 3: Peritoneal deposits
  - Stage 4: Distant metastases
- Overall five year survival is 35%
- Early stage disease has a 70-90% five year survival, but most women present with stage 3 or 4 disease
- Patients who have a reoccurrence often develop chemotherapy resistant disease

OTHER INTERESTING POINTS

- One third of patients with ascites also have a pleural effusion
- This triad of ascites, right sided pleural effusion and ovarian tumour is known as Meig's syndrome
- CA125 can also be raised in fibroids, endometriosis, pregnancy and PID

OTHERS

WILMS' TUMOUR

- Wilms' tumour makes up 6% of childhood malignancies
- 80% occur before the age of 5
- Bilateral or multifocal disease occurs in 5-10%
- It can be associated with mutations of tumour suppressor genes
- Presentation is with an abdominal mass, haematuria and hypertension
- Ultrasound and CT scans are used for diagnosis
- Surgery is the primary treatment
- Post-operative chemotherapy is often needed
- Five year survival ranges from 95% for stage 1 disease to 67% for stage 5
- Even children with pulmonary metastases can be cured (50% with a combination of surgery, chemotherapy and radiotherapy)

PENILE CARCINOMA

- Penile carcinoma is rare, making up less than 1% of male malignancies
- It usually affects the inner prepuce and glans
- 95% are squamous cell carcinomas
- Risk factors include HPV, HIV or genital wart infection, poor local hygiene, smoking and penile injury
- Early circumcision is a protective factor
- Itching or burning under the prepuce is a common initial symptom
- A red area, lump or ulcer then develops
- Inguinal lymphadenopathy occurs in more advanced disease
- Secondary infection may result in purulent discharge
- Metastatic spread can occur, usually to the liver and lungs
- Investigations include biopsy of the primary lesion, FNAC of any enlarged lymph nodes and CT or MRI for staging
- If the biopsy indicates pre-malignant disease, circumcision, and topical agents such as 5-fluorouracil cream is usually the initial treatment
- In invasive disease, surgical excision +/- inguinal lymphadenectomy is performed
- Radiotherapy only has a role in early lesions, particularly in those unfit for surgery
- There is only a limited response to systemic chemotherapy
- The TNM staging system is used
- Overall five year survival is 75%

VAGINAL CANCER

- Vaginal cancer is very rare as a primary cancer, making up less than 2% of gynaecological malignancies
- It tends to affect those aged between 50 and 70 and the risk factors are the same as for cervical cancer
- Most are squamous cell carcinomas and around 5% are adenocarcinoma
- It most commonly affects the posterior wall of the upper third of the vagina and the main presenting feature is blood stained vaginal discharge
- In advanced disease, urinary and rectal symptoms occur as can fistulas
- Treatment depends on the anatomical position and stage, but the mainstay is surgery and radiotherapy
- There is a major role for brachytherapy in the treatment of vaginal cancer, particularly as the affected population are often not fit for surgery
- 5% imiquimod cream may be useful in the treatment of vaginal intraepithelial neoplasia

VULVAL CANCER

- Vulval cancer affects women aged over 50 and makes up just 4% of gynaecological malignancies
- Risk factors include HPV infection, immunosuppression and chronic vulval dystrophy (for example genital herpes, lichen Sclerosis and post radiotherapy)
- Signs and symptoms include itching, pain, ulceration, mass, vaginal discharge or bleeding, dysuria and lymphadenopathy
- 90% are squamous cell carcinomas, which tend to be slow growing
- Melanoma, sarcoma and adenocarcinoma (Bartholin's gland) are other examples
- Investigations include, external genitalia and pelvic examination, biopsy, lymph node FNAC and staging scan
- FIGO stages include: vulval intraepithelial neoplasia (VIN) and stages 1 to 4
- Treatment is primarily surgical; wide local excision or vulvectomy +/- lymph node dissection
- Lymphoedema is a frequent and troublesome complication following inguinal node dissection
- Radiotherapy is used for incomplete clearance and in high risk disease, but chemotherapy has only a minor role
- Stage 1 disease has a 79% five year survival but this is reduced to 13% for stage 4 disease

KEY POINTS SUMMARY

Renal cell carcinoma
- Renal cell carcinoma makes up 3% of all adult cancers
- Classically, patients present with the triad of frank haematuria, loin pain and a loin mass
- Radical nephrectomy is the treatment of choice for localised disease
- Renal tumours are poorly responsive to chemotherapy and radiotherapy, but there is a role for molecular therapy in advanced disease
- Overall five year survival is 40%

Bladder carcinoma
- Bladder carcinoma is the fourth most common cancer in males and eleventh in females
- Painless haematuria is the main presenting complaint in around 90% of patients
- Transitional cell carcinoma is the most common type
- Superficial disease is curable with transurethral resection
- Overall five year survival is 57% for males and 47% for females

Prostate cancer
- Prostate cancer accounts for 15-20% of all male cancers
- 95% of tumours are adenocarcinomas
- Symptoms tend to occur much later than in benign prostatic enlargement
- Surgery and radiotherapy can be a radical treatment for localised disease
- Hormonal manipulation is the mainstay of treatment for metastatic disease
- Overall five year survival is 81%

Testicular cancer
- Testicular cancer is the most common malignancy in men aged 20-40
- The most common presenting feature is a painless mass
- Testicular germ cell tumours are one of the most curable solid malignancies
- Treatment is orchidectomy followed by chemotherapy and/or radiotherapy
- Overall five year survival is 95%

Cervical cancer
- In countries without a screening programme cervical cancer is the second most common cancer cause of death amongst women
- Early cervical cancer is usually asymptomatic, but the most common presenting features are vaginal bleeding or discharge
- Early disease is treated with surgery or radiotherapy, with chemotherapy having a role in more advanced disease
- Overall five year survival is 67%

Endometrial cancer
- Uterine cancer affects more women than does cervical cancer in the UK
- It is very rare before the age of 40 and most commonly presents with abnormal vaginal bleeding
- Most tumours are adenocarcinoma
- The treatment approach tends to be surgery followed by radiotherapy
- Overall five year survival is 80%

Ovarian cancer
- Ovarian cancer is the fifth most common female malignancy
- As it is often asymptomatic or produces vague symptoms in the early stages presentation is often with stage 3 or 4 disease
- Surgery is the mainstay of treatment
- Overall five year survival is 35%

BASAL CELL CARCINOMA

EPIDEMIOLOGY

- Basal cell carcinoma (BCC) is the most common form of skin malignancy
- The incidence is 50-150 per 100,000
- It is more common in males and those aged over 55

RISK FACTORS INCLUDE

- Exposure to ultraviolet radiation from the sun or sunbeds
- It is more chronic exposure experienced by outside workers that is thought to be a risk factor for BCC (and SCC) rather than severe acute exposures as in melanoma
- Fair skinned individuals
- Scarring
- Xeroderma pigmentosum
- Gorlin syndrome (naevoid basal cell carcinoma syndrome)
- Albinism
- Previous radiotherapy
- Immunosuppression
- Previous BCC

SIGNS & SYMPTOMS

- Erythematous patches that may crust or bleed
- The lesion is non-tender, but may be itchy
- It usually affects the sun exposed areas, particularly the head and neck (70% of cases)

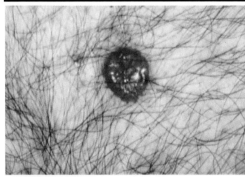

A basal cell carcinoma

INVESTIGATIONS

- Dermatoscopy
- Skin biopsy
- CT if bone involvement is suspected

TYPES/PATHOLOGY/SCREENING

- BCC is a malignancy of the basal cells in the epidermis
- BCCs very rarely metastasise, but they can be destructive of local anatomical structures, especially in the head and neck
- The nodular type have a translucent appearance and may have a central ulcer with an indurated edge (rodent ulcers). They tend to be singular, appear on the face, have telangiectasia and are slow growing
- The superficial type is a scaly plaque most commonly appearing on the trunk or shoulders. They can be multiple
- The pigmented type can be confused with melanoma and is seen more frequently in darker skin types
- The morphoeic type is smooth and flesh coloured and appears similar to a sore. They tend to occur in mid facial sites and are more aggressive. Yellow plaques can form and they may have poorly defined edges

TREATMENT OPTIONS

- Cryosurgery, curettage or electrocautery are only suitable for small BCCs
- Mohs micrographic surgery, where tumours are removed section by section and each one is examined before removing more is preferred by many
- Wide local excision which may require a skin graft or flap
- Radiotherapy is used if surgery isn't possible (but should be avoided in Gorlin syndrome)
- Imiquimod cream can be used for superficial BCCs as it is an immunomodulator
- Fluorouracil 5% cream can also be used, particularly for non facial lesions
- Photodynamic therapy involves the use of a photosensitiser followed by selective exposure to a specific wavelength of light and can be useful for large superficial BCCs

STAGING AND PROGNOSIS

- BCC very rarely requires staging
- Death from BCC is extremely rare, but can occur from sepsis following penetration of the skull or orbit
- There is a significantly higher risk of developing further BCCs that tend to be more resistant to treatment

SQUAMOUS CELL CARCINOMA

EPIDEMIOLOGY

- Squamous cell carcinoma (SCC) is the second most common skin malignancy after basal cell carcinoma
- There are 10,000 new cases in England and Wales each year
- It is more common in males and with advancing age

RISK FACTORS INCLUDE

- Exposure to ultraviolet radiation from the sun or sunbeds
- Ultraviolet B (shortwave) light is more harmful than Ultraviolet A light
- Fair skinned individuals
- Scarring
- Pre-malignant conditions such as solar or actinic keratosis and Bowen's disease can develop into SCC
- Genetic predisposition such as Xeroderma pigmentosum
- Previous radiotherapy
- Immunosuppression
- Leukoplakia

SIGNS & SYMPTOMS

- There is often a tender pink lesion with hard or scaled skin that bleeds easily
- This can develop into a non healing ulcer
- The margins may be rolled
- 70% occur on the head or neck
- Other common sites include the hands, shoulders, arms and legs
- It can rarely develop on the vulva or anus
- As 2% spread systemically, regional lymph nodes should be examined

TYPES/PATHOLOGY/ SCREENING

- SCC is a malignancy of keratinocytes in the epidermis that can also occur in chronic ulcers
- Metastatic risk depends on the presence of the following features
  - Being more than 2mm thick
  - Invasion of the dermis
  - Perineural invasion
  - Occurrence on the ear or lip
  - Poorly differentiated cells

INVESTIGATIONS

- Dermatoscopy
- Skin biopsy
- Lymph node biopsy of any enlarged nodes
- Staging scan in advanced disease or if there are features of metastatic spread

TREATMENT OPTIONS

- Wide local excision, with a 1cm margin
- This may require a skin graft or flap
- Lymph node clearance in cases of spread
- Radiotherapy is an effective adjuvant treatment in high risk SCCs
- Radiotherapy can also be used in those that are not fit for surgery
- Curettage, electrodesiccation or cryosurgery can be considered for small lesions
- Immunotherapy; interferon can be used in metastatic disease

STAGING AND PROGNOSIS

- The TNM staging system is used initially and then classified into stages 1-4
- Overall five year survival is 98%
- 2% metastasise, and these patients have a 30% five year survival

OTHER INTERESTING POINTS

- Bowen's disease is a pre-malignant skin condition (carcinoma in situ), that can be found on a lower leg, typically in older women
- Bowen's disease can also appear on mucous membranes and develop into squamous cell carcinoma
- This is often treated with fluorouracil cream

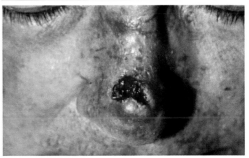

A squamous cell carcinoma

MELANOMA

EPIDEMIOLOGY

- Melanomas make up 2.5% of all malignancies
- It has an overall annual incidence of 1.5 to 4 per 100,000, ranging from 0.7 for black Americans to 40 for white Australians
- The incidence has been increasing over recent years at a rate of 50% per decade
- It is more common in males than females, and peaks in the fifth decade of life

RISK FACTORS INCLUDE

- Recurrent, acute, significant sun exposure, particularly in childhood
- Fair skinned, freckled people and red hair types
- A high number of common naevi
- The presence of solar keratosis and atypical moles (dysplastic naevus)
- Family or previous personal history of melanoma

SIGNS & SYMPTOMS

- A 'mole' that is enlarging with an irregular border, changing shape or colour, is tender or itchy and is bleeding or inflamed
- In males, melanomas are most common on the back or trunk but in females, they are more common on the legs
- Lymphadenopathy near the melanoma site

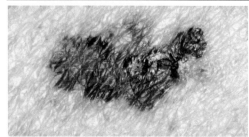

A melanoma, with an irregular border and different colours within it

INVESTIGATIONS

- Dermatoscopy
- Skin biopsy, preferably excisional
- Lymph node needle aspiration or sentinel lymph node biopsy
- CT scan if metastases are suspected
- Routine bloods, particularly FBC, LFTs and LDH

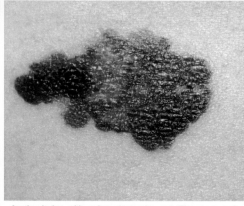

Another lesion, with an irregular border, and different areas of colour suggestion melanoma

TYPES/PATHOLOGY/ SCREENING

- Melanoma is a neoplasm of the epidermal melanocytes
- The superficial spreading type makes up 70% of melanomas. They usually arise from a pre-existing naevus and have an initial radial growth phase (horizontal plane) and tend to affect those aged 40-60
- Nodular melanoma makes up 15% of cases of melanoma and are fast growing dark coloured, raised (or dome shaped) lesions most often found on the chest or back. They tend to arise from previously normal skin and are more aggressive than the superficial spreading type
- Lentigo maligna melanoma makes up 5-10% of cases and develops from a previous lentigo maligna on sun exposed areas in the elderly (usually females). This type is a slow growing pigmented area of skin that is flat and grows outwards giving it a much better prognosis. If it becomes nodular, this is a poor prognostic sign
- Acral lentiginous melanoma is rare in Caucasians and tends to affect African or Asian races on the palms of hands, soles of feet and under the nails
- Amelanotic melanoma are rare pigment lacking melanomas and as such are difficult to diagnose
- Common metastatic sites are the lungs, liver, bone, brain, abdomen and lymph nodes
- There is no national screening programme
- The public are advised to regularly check their own skin for melanoma, especially pre-existing moles and to look for any new changes

MELANOMA

TREATMENT OPTIONS

- Wide local excision, which may require skin grafts or local flaps
- Lymph node dissection if confirmed involvement of lymph nodes
- Metastasectomy if possible
- Chemotherapy has a poor response rate (around 20%)
- Dacarbazine is the most common single agent used
- This can be combined with carbomustine, vinblastine, cisplatin or temozolomide in aggressive metastatic disease
- Biological therapy such as ipilimumab, vemurafenib interferon alpha and interleukin 2 have received much attention due to the poor response to chemotherapy
- Radiotherapy has a very limited role
- Protection from further sun exposure and the teaching of self examination to reduce future recurrence is important

STAGING AND PROGNOSIS

- The TNM system is the most specific staging used
- T uses the Breslow depth (an important indicator of prognosis) and the presence of ulceration
- N takes into account micrometastasis, macrometastasis and satellite metastasis
- M specifies whether spread is to other areas of skin or nodes, the lungs, or other organs
- Overall five year survival in the UK is 85% for females and 73% for males, but is drastically different depending upon the stage
- 8% of patients with melanoma develop a second melanoma within two years of diagnosis
- There can be a time lag of 20 years between resection of a primary lesion to the development of metastases
- Up to 20% of patients develop CNS metastases

KEY POINTS SUMMARY

Basal cell carcinoma
- Basal cell carcinoma is the most common form of skin malignancy
- The key risk factors are related to a chronic exposure to ultraviolet light
- Around 70% occur on the head and neck and 90% are of the nodular and superficial types
- Treatment options include excision, radiotherapy, topical therapy and photodynamic therapy
- Due to the low metastatic potential, death is extremely rare from basal cell carcinoma

Squamous cell carcinoma
- Squamous cell carcinoma is the second most common form of skin malignancy
- It occurs on sun exposed areas and most commonly affects the head and neck
- Squamous cell carcinoma can occur at sites of scars, chronic inflammation, ulceration and in wounds
- Squamous cell carcinoma has a higher propensity for recurrence and metastatic spread than basal cell carcinoma
- Wide local excision is the treatment of choice
- Overall five year survival is 98%

Melanoma
- Melanoma makes up 2.5% of all malignancies and the incidence is increasing
- A greater percentage of younger adults are affected by melanoma than basal cell or squamous cell carcinomas
- 85% of cases are superficial or nodular in type
- In the absence of lymphadenopathy, the Breslow depth and presence of ulceration are the key prognostic indicators
- Surgery is the treatment of choice
- Melanoma tends to be resistant to chemotherapy and so there has been great interest in biological therapies
- There can be a long lag between initial treatment and the occurrence of metastases
- Overall five year survival is 85% for females and 73% for males

BRAIN TUMOURS

EPIDEMIOLOGY

- Primary brain tumours make up around 1.5% of malignancies diagnosed in the UK
- However, brain metastases are the most common cause of intracranial malignancy
- In patients with a systemic malignancy, around 10% will develop brain metastases
- Brain tumours can occur at any age, but are most common in those aged 60-75
- Primary tumours are more commonly seen in patients from higher social classes, but the reverse trend is seen for brain metastases
- Benign tumours are more common in females, but malignant tumours are more common in males

RISK FACTORS INCLUDE

- Ionising radiation
- Genetic conditions including tuberous sclerosis, neurofibromatosis, Li-Fraumeni syndrome, Von Hippel-Lindau syndrome and Turner syndrome
- Previous malignancy
- Family history of a brain tumour in a first degree relative
- Immunosuppression, particularly HIV
- Environmental factors such as vinyl chloride

SIGNS & SYMPTOMS

- Signs and symptoms are due to local brain invasion, compression of adjacent structures and raised intracranial pressure
- The clinical manifestation depends on the site of the tumour as well as the rate of growth
- Headache, usually an early morning headache that is dull and constant
- Seizures
- Nausea and vomiting
- Cognitive decline
- Ataxia
- Behavioural change
- Dysarthria
- Aphasia
- Syncope
- Hypertension
- Bradycardia (Cushing's reflex)
- Papilloedema
- Reduced level of consciousness
- Stroke
- Other focal neurology such as diplopia, visual field deficits and limb weakness

SCREENING/TYPES/ PATHOLOGY

- Brain tumours are a heterogeneous group of lesions that can be classified by their tissue of origin:
- Neuroepithelial tissue (gliomas, that make up around 60% of brain tumours):
  - Astrocytomas, which include glioblastoma multiforme
  - Oligodendroglial tumours
  - Ependymal tumours
  - Mixed (gangliocytomas, oligoastrocytomas)
  - Choroid plexus tumours
- Meninges:
  - Meningioma
  - Mesenchymal tumours
  - Melanocytoma
- Cranial nerves:
  - Schwannoma
  - Neurofibroma
  - Malignant peripheral nerve sheath tumour
- Germ cell tumours such as embryonal carcinoma
- Sellar tumours such as craniopharyngioma
- Others, including haemangioblastomas and lymphomas

INVESTIGATIONS

- Full neurological examination
- Biochemical and endocrine profile
- CT scan
- MRI is more sensitive
- MRA (magnetic resonance angiography) and MRS (magnetic resonance spectroscopy) can sometimes provide additional useful information
- A PET scan can help determine the grade of a tumour
- Lumbar puncture
- Biopsy and/or surgical exploration
- Investigations to look for a primary tumour

STAGING AND PROGNOSIS

- Tumours are graded according to their aggressiveness with the WHO grade
- Grade 1 is slow growing, whereas grade 4 is very aggressive
- Five year survival is 15%, but prognosis depends upon histology, grade, size and location of the tumour and age at diagnosis

BRAIN TUMOURS

TREATMENT OPTIONS

General
- Multidisciplinary team discussion
- Symptom control such as the use of anti-epileptics

Primary tumours
- Surgery is the treatment of choice whenever possible
- Surgery can also be used to provide palliation by relieving pressure symptoms and treating hydrocephalus
- Radiotherapy can prolong survival following surgery for high grade tumours
- Radiotherapy may also be used as a primary treatment
- Stereotactic/gamma knife radiosurgery is a relatively new option and is only available at certain centres in the UK
- Chemotherapy has a limited role

Brain metastases
- Corticosteroids are useful in the acute setting to reduce surrounding oedema
- Surgery is only suitable for a small number of young, fit patients with a low number of metastases
- Stereotactic radiosurgery may again be an option
- Radiotherapy however is the most frequently used treatment modality
- Whole brain palliative radiotherapy can improve symptoms in around three-quarters of patients
- Chemotherapy can have a role if the primary cancer is chemosensitive such as in haematological malignancies and small cell lung cancer

BRAIN METASTASES

- The most common origins of brain metastases are lung, breast, colorectal, melanoma and kidney
- The route of spread is mostly haematogenous
- This means that the location of metastases is normally between the grey and white matter where cerebral blood vessels narrow and tumour cells nest (also known as the 'watershed' areas)
- Clinical presentation is similar to that of primary brain tumours
- Management is covered above
- Prognosis varies and can depend upon the primary malignancy

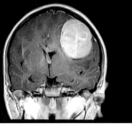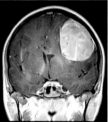

A large tumour causing midline shift

SPECIFIC TUMOURS

Astrocytoma
- Astrocytomas are the most common form of primary brain tumour
- The grade is very important in determining treatment and prognosis

Glioblastoma multiforme
- Glioblastoma multiforme is an aggressive astrocytoma (WHO grade 4)
- Treatment involves debulking surgery and radiotherapy
- NICE recommends temozolomide and carmustine implants
- Systemic chemotherapy can also be used
- Prognosis is poor with a 6% five year survival

Ependymoma
- Ependymomas make up 5% of gliomas
- They arise from ependymal cells which line the ventricles and spinal cord
- Treatment is with surgery and radiotherapy, with chemotherapy for recurrences
- Prognosis is better than the brain tumour average with a 50% five year survival

Meningioma
- Meningiomas make up 25% of brain tumours
- Previous radiation is a significant risk factor
- They are benign and slow growing but can still cause significant morbidity and mortality
- They are most common in elderly women
- Treatment is with surgery and/or radiotherapy
- There is a 60-80% five year survival

Pituitary adenoma
- Pituitary adenomas make up 15% of brain tumours
- They are almost always benign
- They can be secretary and result in excess production of hormones
- Medical treatment is used for the endocrine symptoms, but surgery may be needed if there are pressure or visual symptoms
- Five year survival is 85%

OSTEOSARCOMA

EPIDEMIOLOGY

- Osteosarcoma makes up 0.2% of all cancers in the UK
- The incidence is 0.7 per 100,000
- 75% occur in those aged under 20 years of age
- It is the most common primary malignancy of bone in children and adolescents
- There is a second peak in incidence in over 65s (due to Paget's disease, infarcts and previous radiotherapy)
- It is more common in males

RISK FACTORS INCLUDE

- In children and adolescents, the majority of cases are sporadic
- In older patients, Paget disease (due to the risk of sarcomatous transformation) is a major risk factor
- Benign bone lesions
- Previous chemotherapy or radiotherapy
- Genetic conditions such as
- Hereditary retinoblastoma
- Li-Fraumeni syndrome (mutation in p53)
- Rothmund-Thomson syndrome

SIGNS & SYMPTOMS

- Localised pain and swelling, often around the knee for a number of months
- The most common sites are the femur, tibia and humerus
- There may be a limp
- Constitutional symptoms are less common

TYPES/PATHOLOGY/SCREENING

- Osteosarcoma occurs in the metaphyses of long bones
- It is a primary malignant tumour of the bone characterised by production of osteoid or immature bone by a sarcomatous stroma
- The peak incidence in adolescence is due to the 'growth spurt'
- Tumours can be osteoblastic, chondroblastic or fibroblastic. Other rare types include small cell, telangiectatic and multifocal
- The most common site of metastasis is the lungs, which can occur rapidly (10-20% at presentation)

INVESTIGATIONS

- Plain radiographs may show destruction of the normal trabecular bone pattern, indistinct margins and periosteal new bone formation, lifting off the cortex (Codman's triangle)
- Raised ALP and LDH
- Biopsy
- Immunohistochemistry to confirm diagnosis
- MRI of entire long bone for surgical planning
- Chest x-ray and CT thorax for metastases
- PET/CT for multiple lesions

TREATMENT OPTIONS

- Multidisciplinary team discussion including a thoracic surgeon in cases of lung metastases
- Surgical resection can be limb sparing for tumours in the extremities. This often involves a prosthesis
- Amputation if limb sparing is not possible, following post-operative infections or if major neurovascular structures are involved
- Neo-adjuvant (if a limb saving procedure is planned) and adjuvant chemotherapy
- Regimes often include methotrexate with folinic acid or cisplatin with doxorubicin
- Radiotherapy is only used when there is no surgical option or for small cell osteosarcoma

STAGING AND PROGNOSIS

- The Musculoskeletal Tumour Society (MSTS) Staging (Enneking) system is used
- Stage
  - I - low grade
  - II - high grade
  - III - distant metastases
- Anatomy
  - A - intra-compartmental (contained within the bone cortex)
  - B - extra-compartmental
- Overall five year survival is 40%
- 65% of those with extremity tumours can expect long term survival, but this reduces to 20% in those with metastatic disease

OTHER INTERESTING POINTS

- In the 1970s, 90% of osteosarcoma patients would progress despite achieving local tumour control, but survival rates have improved due to the effective use of chemotherapy

SOFT TISSUE SARCOMA

EPIDEMIOLOGY

- Soft tissue sarcoma collectively accounts for 1% of all malignancies and 12-15% of paediatric malignancies diagnosed annually in the UK
- The majority of cases of adult soft tissue sarcoma are in those aged over 50, but it can affect any age
- The incidence has increased over last 20 years but this is most likely due to improved diagnosis and reporting

TYPES/PATHOLOGY/ SCREENING

- It is not common to have constitutional symptoms and benign masses are far more common, and hence diagnosis is often delayed
- The department of health have therefore published these criteria for primary care physicians to prompt urgent referral
- Soft tissue mass larger than 5cm
- Painful lump
- Lump that is growing
- Lump of any size deep to the muscle fascia
- Lump recurrence after previous excision
- Soft tissue sarcomas are a heterogeneous group of tumours of mesenchymal origin
- Embryonic mesenchymal cells are pluripotent, hence the histological spectrum of soft tissue sarcomas involves over fifty morphological subtypes
- These are some of the most common:
- Gastrointestinal stroma (GIST)
- Undifferentiated pleomorphic sarcoma
- Adipose tissue (liposarcoma)
- Smooth muscle (leiomyosarcoma)
- Synovium (synovial sarcoma)
- Nerve sheaths (malignant peripheral nerve sheath tumour)
- Skeletal (rhabdomyosarcoma)
- Fibrous tissue (fibrosarcoma)
- Blood vessels (angiosarcoma)
- There is a tendency to grow along tissue planes
- They have a haematogenous route of spread, primarily to the lungs
- The probability of metastatic spread is 50% in high grade sarcomas compared with just 15% in low grade sarcomas
- Occasionally spread occurs to regional lymph nodes (a poor prognostic factor)
- The Trojani grading system is often used

RISK FACTORS INCLUDE

- Almost all are de novo
- Genetic predisposition
- Li-Fraumeni syndrome
- Neurofibromatosis type 1
- Gardiner's syndrome
- Von Hippel-Lindau syndrome
- Hereditary retinoblastoma
- Previous chemotherapy or radiotherapy
- Chemical carcinogens
- Chronic irritation and lymphoedema
- Viruses, such as Kaposi's sarcoma

SIGNS & SYMPTOMS

- A gradually enlarging painless mass
- Pain is an indicator of a poor prognosis
- Specific symptoms depend upon the site, but may include abdominal pain, neurological symptoms, haematuria, abnormal uterine bleeding, and nasal obstruction and/or bleeding
- Paraesthesia or oedema in an affected limb
- They can occur anywhere but the most common sites are
- Thigh, buttock or groin
- Torso
- Upper extremity
- Retroperitoneum
- Head and neck

INVESTIGATIONS

- Plain radiography is useful to rule out bony origins
- MRI is the preferred imaging modality
- CT however can still have a role looking for pulmonary metastases and for retroperitoneal sarcomas
- The presence or absence of pulmonary metastases affects management
- PET is only useful in high grade tumours
- Biopsy (most often core needle) for morphological pattern, immunohistochemical staining and fluorescent in situ hybridization (FISH) and reverse transcriptase PCR
- Core needle biopsy is preferred to FNAC due to low sensitivity and specificity associated with the latter
- Follow up should include chest x-rays for distant pulmonary metastases and CT scanning in visceral or retroperitoneal disease

SOFT TISSUE SARCOMA

TREATMENT OPTIONS

- Multidisciplinary team discussion
- Surgical resection by wide local excision is the mainstay of treatment
- Reconstruction may be required following very wide excision
- Pulmonary metastectomy may be possible in selected patients
- Radiotherapy can be neo-adjuvant or adjuvant in high grade sarcomas over 5cm or if resection is incomplete
- Radiotherapy can also be used in the palliative setting particularly in those not fit for surgery
- Chemotherapy as adjuvant therapy is only usually used in those with a high risk of recurrence or symptomatic metastatic disease as its role in primary treatment is debatable due to lack of good evidence that it gives a clear survival benefit
- An example regime would include doxorubicin with ifosfamide

STAGING AND PROGNOSIS

- Not applicable to all soft tissue sarcomas
- The most widely used is the TNM system in combination with the histological grade
  - 1 Well differentiated, low grade
  - 2 Moderately differentiated
  - 3 Poorly differentiated, high grade
- Overall five year survival is 51%, but depends on location, size, depth, grade and metastases
- Patients with a low grade, superficial tumour or a tumour less than 5cm can expect a 90% five year survival

OTHER INTERESTING POINTS

- Peripheral nerves are actually ectodermal in origin but malignant nerve sheath tumours behave similarly to soft tissue sarcomas, hence are included in the classification

OTHERS

EWING'S SARCOMA

- Ewing's sarcoma is a small round cell tumour primarily affecting bone in children and adolescents (it can rarely occur in soft tissues)
- It occurs as a result of a translocation between chromosomes 11 and 22
- Incidence is 0.2 per 100,000 (30 a year in the UK)
- It is more common in males and most occur between the ages of 10 and 15
- It is very uncommon in African and Asian populations
- Signs and symptoms include fever, anaemia, leucocytosis, malaise, weight loss and pain and swelling at the tumour site
- The most commonly affected sites are the pelvis, long bones, ribs and spine
- There is a higher proportion of axial involvement compared to osteosarcoma
- Combined chemotherapy, surgery and radiotherapy is the preferred approach, most often in that order
- Adjuvant multi-drug chemotherapy can be used
- There is a 50-70% five year survival for localised disease, but is 10-20% in metastatic disease

GASTROINTESTINAL STROMAL TUMOUR

- Gastrointestinal stromal tumours (GISTs) are a rare type of sarcoma occurring in the stomach (60%), small intestine (25%) or colon/rectum (10%)
- GISTs have an over-expression of a CD117 surface receptor due to a defect in the c-kit gene
- Incidence is 1-2 per 100,000
- 75% occur in those aged over 50
- The risk of occurrence is increased in neurofibromatosis
- Symptoms include abdominal pain, early satiety, bloating, vomiting +/- haematemesis, melaena, fresh PR bleeding, fever, weight loss and night sweats
- Surgery can be curative
- Biological therapy such as imatinib (a tyrosine kinase inhibitor) is useful in those who are CD117 positive
- Sunitinib can be used second line
- There is a 64% five year survival when disease is organ confined, but just a 13% five year survival in metastatic disease, despite spread outside of the abdominal cavity being unusual

OTHERS

CHONDROSARCOMA

- Chondrosarcoma is a malignant bone sarcoma that produces chondroid matrix
- They are the second most common sarcoma affecting bone, after osteosarcoma
- It mostly affects those aged 40-60 years
- They can arise from pre-existing chondromas or osteochondromas or be of primary origin
- 90% are slow growing with low probability of metastatic spread and the other 10% are high grade but are more responsive to treatment
- The key complaint is of a deep dull pain with swelling
- They can present with a pathological fracture
- The most commonly affected sites are the proximal femur, pelvis and proximal humerus
- Surgery is the only chance of a cure
- Intralesional curettage can be performed for confined disease
- Radiotherapy can be used in incomplete excisions or for palliation
- Chemotherapy is only occasionally used
- Overall five year survival is 48-60%

RHABDOMYOSARCOMA

- Rhabdomyosarcoma is the most common soft tissue tumour in children
- There are around 60 cases a year in the UK
- 87% occur in those aged under 15 years
- Most are sporadic but some are associated with familial syndromes
- They come from skeletal muscle lineage
- There are 4 subtypes, the most common of which is embryonal, which is the most treatable and carries the best prognosis
- The other subtypes are alveolar, botryoid and pleomorphic
- The most common locations are head and neck (40%) genitourinary (20%) and muscles, limbs, chest and abdominal wall (20%)
- Symptoms are related to the site of the tumour but also to the metastatic site, most commonly lung, bone, omentum and pleura
- Primary treatment is surgery
- Neo-adjuvant or adjuvant chemotherapy is used for cytoreduction and eradication of metastases
- Radiotherapy can be used to control local residual disease post operatively
- Chemotherapy and radiotherapy increase cure rates; with combined therapy 70% of children with localised disease can be cured
- In metastatic disease five year survival is 30%

KAPOSI'S SARCOMA

- Kaposi's sarcoma is an angioproliferative sarcoma that requires infection with HHV-8 (human herpes virus 8) for it's development
- There are 4 clinical types:
1. Classic (or sporadic) affects those aged over 60 in the Mediterranean and Eastern Europe, has a 3:1 male:female ratio and most frequently affects the lower limbs
2. Endemic (or African) classically affects male adults and children with a normal immune system near to the African equator
3. Iatrogenic (or transplant related) is common in those with solid organ transplants and with the use of ciclosporin
4. Epidemic (or AIDS associated) may regress with effective HIV treatment
- Macules, plaques and nodules form on the skin. These may be red, purple, brown or black and can ulcerate and bleed
- Localised lymphoedema can also occur
- Oral and gastrointestinal tract mucosal involvement can result in bleeding or diarrhoea
- Pulmonary involvement results in dyspnoea, cough and possible haemoptysis
- Biopsy, HIV testing and CD4 counts are the key investigations
- It is incurable
- The primary approach is to treat the underlying cause
- Specific treatments depend upon the number of lesions and immunological status
- Advice regarding camouflage make up should be given
- Local radiotherapy, chemotherapy (systemic or intralesional) can be effective, but effects are temporary
- Surgery may be required for complications of gastrointestinal lesions
- There is an indolent course, but occasionally a rapidly progressive course occurs
- Advanced pulmonary involvement has a prognosis of less than six months

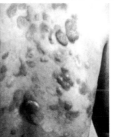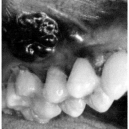

The appearance of Kaposi's sarcoma

KEY POINTS SUMMARY

Overall
- Sarcomas are a very heterogeneous group of tumours that can arise from any cell of mesenchymal origin
- They are named based on the type of tissue the tumour most resembles
- Each subtype behaves and responds to treatment differently
- Sarcomas are normally graded based on their cellular differentiation
- The most common site of metastases is the lung, the presence of which significantly worsens prognosis
- Surgery remains the most important treatment modality but the introduction of chemotherapy has vastly improved survival rates for most sarcomas

Osteosarcoma
- Osteosarcoma is the most common primary malignancy of bone in children and adolescents
- There is a second peak of incidence in those aged over 65
- Presentation is usually with localised pain for several months with a mass found on examination
- Primary treatment is surgical, which may be limb salvaging or may require an amputation, with adjuvant or neo-adjuvant chemotherapy
- Overall five year survival is 40%

Soft tissue sarcoma
- Soft tissue sarcomas make up around 1% of all malignancies
- They are a heterogeneous group of tumours of mesenchymal origin, having more than fifty different histological subtypes
- The most common presenting feature is a slow growing painless mass
- MRI is the preferred imaging modality
- Surgery is the mainstay of treatment
- Radiotherapy may also be used, but chemotherapy has not been shown to demonstrate a clear survival benefit
- Overall five year survival is 51%

Ewing's sarcoma
- Ewing's sarcoma is a small round cell tumour primary bone tumour that most commonly affects children and adolescents
- It occurs as a result of a translocation between chromosomes 11 and 22
- There is a higher proportion of axial involvement compared to osteosarcoma

Gastrointestinal stromal tumour
- Gastrointestinal stromal tumours most frequently affect the stomach
- Surgery can be curative and there is a role for tyrosine kinase inhibitors

Kaposi's sarcoma
- Kaposi's sarcoma requires infection with human herpes virus 8 for it's development
- It is incurable and often runs an indolent course
- Treatment is aimed at symptoms and the underlying cause

Chondrosarcoma
- Chondrosarcoma is the second most common sarcoma affecting bone, after osteosarcoma
- Surgery can offer a chance of cure

Rhabdomyosarcoma
- Rhabdomyosarcoma is the most common soft tissue tumour in children
- Combined therapy can produce cure rates of 70% in children with localised disease

HODGKIN'S LYMPHOMA

EPIDEMIOLOGY

- Hodgkin's lymphoma makes up 6.5% of all haematological malignancies
- Incidence is 2.8 per 100,000 in the UK (1500 new cases per year)
- The are two peaks of incidence; ages 20-30 and 70-80

RISK FACTORS INCLUDE

- Socioeconomic status and environmental factors; a high standard of living is associated with developing nodular sclerosis
- Infective agents, especially EBV
- Immunosuppression such as HIV or following an organ transplant
- Autoimmune disorders
- Familial risk (HLA-A1 and HLA-A12)

SIGNS & SYMPTOMS

- Painless localised lymphadenopathy
- The lymphadenopathy is most commonly cervical or supraclavicular (70%), but also axillary (20%) and inguinal (10%)
- Incidental mediastinal mass on chest x-ray
- B symptoms:
  - Fever over 38°C
  - Unintentional weight loss (more than 10% in 6 months)
  - Sweats (drenching and nocturnal)
- Other constitutional symptoms such as fatigue and pruritus
- Repeated infections
- Persistent cough
- Splenomegaly
- Alcohol induced pain is rare (less than 10%) but specific
- Occasionally, features of paraneoplastic syndromes occur

INVESTIGATIONS

- Blood tests: FBC, U&Es, LFTs, LDH, ESR, β microglobulin and viral screen
- Chest x-ray (for mediastinal adenopathy)
- CT neck, thorax, abdomen and pelvis
- PET scan to differentiate between scar tissue and lymphoma
- Lymph node biopsy is necessary for diagnosis (the presence of Reed-Sternberg cells in an inflammatory background)
- Bone marrow biopsy looking for bone marrow infiltration (1 in 25 at diagnosis)
- Staging laparotomy is no longer performed

TYPES/PATHOLOGY/ SCREENING

- Hodgkin's lymphoma arises from germinal centres or post-germinal centre B cells and has a unique cellular composition
- The majority of cells are inflammatory and a minority are neoplastic cells (Reed-Sternberg cells, see left)
- There are two forms of Hodgkin's Lymphoma
- The classical type includes
  - Nodular sclerosis (most common, 70%)
  - Mixed cellularity (10%)
  - Lymphocyte rich (best prognosis, 15%)
  - Lymphocyte deplete (worse prognosis, 5%)
- Nodular lymphocyte predominant is the other form, where cells retain immunophenotypic features of germinal centre B cells
- This form is less common and more indolent

STAGING AND PROGNOSIS

- The Ann Arbor Staging system is used
- I. Involves one group of lymph nodes
- II. Involves two or more groups of lymph nodes on the same side of the diaphragm
- III. Involves two or more groups of lymph nodes on both sides of the diaphragm
- IV. Involves metastases to the liver, bone or lungs
- A. No B symptoms
- B. B symptoms present
- Most relapses occur in the first two years following initial therapy
- Overall there is an 80% five year survival in the UK
- Stage 1 and 2 disease has a 91-94% five year survival, stage 3 and 4 disease has a 59-90% five year survival

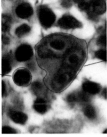

Normal lymphocyte

Reed-Sternberg Cell

Hodgkin's lymphoma is characterised by Reed-Sternberg cells, which are multinucleated giant cells of B cell origin

HODGKIN'S LYMPHOMA

TREATMENT OPTIONS

- Multidisciplinary team discussion
- Vaccinations
- Stage I and II with no B symptoms is treated with a short course of chemotherapy followed by 4 to 6 weeks of radiotherapy
- Stage IB and IIB to IVB is treated with combination chemotherapy and radiotherapy
- The most common chemotherapy regime is 4 to 8 cycles of ABVD (doxorubicin (adriamycin), bleomycin, vinblastine and dacarbazine)
- ABVD is the gold standard and has replaced old regimes such as MOPP due to reduced side effects such as infertility and secondary malignancies
- Radiotherapy is usually targeted to a focused area of lymph nodes
- Steroids can have a role in advanced stages
- Biological therapies such as rituximab can be used for nodular lymphocyte predominant lymphoma
- Bone marrow or stem cell transplant for recurrences or drug resistant disease

OTHER INTERESTING POINTS

- Early exposure to common infections can be protective in ones risk of developing Hodgkin's Lymphoma
- Since the 1970's the incidence in females has increased by around 20%, but the incidence in males has remained static
- It is estimated that 40% of cases in the UK are related to EBV infection
- Factors indicating poor prognosis include an increased stage of disease, B symptoms, age over 40, mediastinal bulk adenopathy and the lymphocyte depleted histological type
- More than half of Hodgkin's lymphoma deaths are in those aged over 65
- With survival increasing, the incidence of secondary malignancies is more important
- Common secondary malignancies include acute myeloid leukaemia, non-Hodgkin's lymphomas and lung, colorectal and breast cancers. Hence patients are monitored closely and begin screening at a younger age

NON-HODGKIN'S LYMPHOMA

EPIDEMIOLOGY

- Non-Hodgkin's lymphoma is more than five times more common than Hodgkin's lymphoma
- It makes up 44% of all haematological malignancies
- Incidence is 15 per 100,000 in the UK (9700 new cases per year)
- Incidence increases with age

Malignant B-cell lymphocytes in Burkitt's lymphoma

TYPES/PATHOLOGY/ SCREENING

- Non Hodgkin's lymphoma is a diverse group of malignant neoplasms derived from B and T cells, their progenitors or natural killer cells
- Histological classification is complicated, but types can be divided by grade
- Low grade disease is slow growing and presentation is often delayed
- Examples include
- Follicular lymphoma (B cell lymphoma)
- Mantle cell (behaves aggressively despite being low grade)
- Splenic marginal zone lymphoma
- MALT lymphoma (B cell lymphoma common in the stomach)
- High grade disease is fast growing and early intervention and treatment is important
- Examples include
- Diffuse large B cell lymphoma (constitutes a third of all non-Hodgkin's lymphomas)
- Diffuse mixed cell lymphoma
- Burkitt's lymphoma
- Anaplastic large cell lymphoma

NON-HODGKIN'S LYMPHOMA

RISK FACTORS INCLUDE

- Immunosuppression such as post organ transplant, HIV and autoimmune disorders
- Viruses:
  - EBV increases the incidence of Burkitt's lymphoma
  - Human T cell lymphoma virus 1 (HTLV1)
  - Hepatitis C
  - Human herpes simplex virus (HSV-6)
  - Helicobacter pylori can increase the risk of MALT (mucosa associated lymphoid tissue) lymphoma
- Coeliac disease (T cell intestinal lymphoma)
- Family history (bcl gene expression and 14:8 translocations)
- Previous Hodgkin's lymphoma or leukaemia

SIGNS & SYMPTOMS

- Depends upon the location and type of lymphoma
- High grade lymphoma presents with a rapidly growing mass and B symptoms
- Low grade lymphoma can present with slow growing lymphadenopathy, symptoms of cytopenias, hepatosplenomegaly and frequent infections
- The neck is the most common site of lymphadenopathy
- Gastrointestinal tract lymphoma may present with weight loss, nausea and vomiting, abdominal mass and occasionally bowel obstruction or perforation
- Central nervous system (CNS) lymphoma may present with headache, focal neurological signs, seizures, paralysis or spinal cord compression

INVESTIGATIONS

- An FBC may show anaemia, leukopenia and thrombocytopenia
- LDH, ESR, calcium, urate and other routine biochemistry
- Serum protein electrophoresis may show a monoclonal band
- Chest x-ray
- CT neck, thorax, abdomen and pelvis investigating the extent of disease
- Lymph node biopsy
- PET in high grade tumours
- Bone marrow aspirate and trephine biopsy
- Lumbar puncture for CNS involvement
- Endoscopy for mucosal involvement

TREATMENT OPTIONS

- Multidisciplinary team discussion
- Vaccinations
- Low grade disease is treated with radiotherapy, and chemotherapy (such as R-CVP; rituximab, cyclophosphamide, vincristine and prednisolone)
- Interferon α has a role in advanced stage low grade disease
- Chemotherapy is the primary treatment in high grade disease
- RCHOP (rituximab, cyclophosphamide, doxorubicin, vincristine, prednisolone) is a frequently used regime
- CNS prophylaxis with intrathecal methotrexate in high risk patients
- Radiotherapy can have a role in high grade disease, particularly in those with areas of initial high bulk or those too frail for chemotherapy
- Bone marrow transplant may be considered if there is a high likelihood of recurrence or previous failed treatments

STAGING AND PROGNOSIS

- Staging is the same as in Hodgkin's Lymphoma, but can be simplified into the following
  - Limited disease: stage I or II with no B symptoms
  - Advanced disease: stage III or IV, a tumour bigger than 10cm or any B symptoms
- The overall ten year survival rate in the UK is 51%
- Poor prognostic factors include age over 60 at time of diagnosis, stage III or IV at diagnosis, raised LDH and poor performance status

OTHER INTERESTING POINTS

- Non-Hodgkin's lymphoma is more frequently disseminated at diagnosis than Hodgkin's disease
- Richter's transformation is the term used when a low grade lymphoma (or chronic lymphocytic leukaemia) transforms into a high grade lymphoma (most commonly diffuse large B cell lymphoma)
- Mycosis fungoides is a rare cutaneous T cell lymphoma. It is low grade and can often be treated with ultraviolet light.

ACUTE MYELOID LEUKAEMIA

EPIDEMIOLOGY

- Acute myeloid leukaemia (AML) is the most common acute leukaemia in adults
- There are around 2200 new cases in the UK each year
- The median age of diagnosis is 65 and it is slightly more common in males

RISK FACTORS INCLUDE

- Radiation from previous radiotherapy or post radioactive warfare
- Benzene exposure in pollution and smoking
- Genetic disorders such as Down's syndrome Fanconi's anaemia, and Bloom's syndrome
- Previous chemotherapy
- A pre-existing haematological disorder (myelodysplastic or myeloproliferative)
- Auto-immune conditions such as rheumatoid arthritis

SIGNS & SYMPTOMS

- Fatigue, lethargy and weakness
- Frequent infections
- Bruising or bleeding, particularly gingival bleeding, epistaxis, or menorrhagia
- Dizziness
- Dyspnoea
- Fever
- Weight loss
- Arthralgia
- Pallor and petechiae
- Hepatomegaly
- Splenomegaly
- Gingivitis
- Examination of the ocular fundus reveals haemorrhages and/or whitish plaques in most patients
- Patients may also present with biochemical abnormalities

INVESTIGATIONS

- An FBC will typically show a large number of blasts with depleted neutrophils, anaemia and thrombocytopenia
- Other blood tests including a blood film, U&Es, LFTs, bone profile, clotting screen LDH, urate and viral screen
- Bone marrow aspiration and trephine
- Tissue typing (HLA matching) if a bone marrow transplant is a possibility
- PCR and immunophenotyping

TYPES/PATHOLOGY/ SCREENING

- AML is a haemopoietic malignancy involving precursor cells of the myeloid line that are progenitors of monocytes, granulocytes, erythrocytes and megakaryocytes
- There is an accumulation of blasts (immature cells) in the bone marrow and blood
- The bone marrow is often so hypercellular with blasts that it has very few normal cellular components remaining
- Auer rods are pathognomonic of myeloblasts and sometimes clump into Auer bodies
- Classification is using either the French-American-British (FAB) classification system or the WHO system
- The FAB system has 8 types from M0 to M7
  - The most common (more than 50%) are M0-M2 which are all myeloblastic leukaemias
  - M3 (acute promyelocytic leukaemia) makes up 10% of cases
  - M4 (acute myelomonocytic leukaemia) makes up 20% of cases
  - M5 (acute monocytic leukaemia) makes up 15% of cases
  - M6 (acute erythroleukaemia) and M7 (acute megakaryocytic leukaemia) are very rare
- The newer WHO classification, which is now superseding the original FAB system is based upon a combination of morphology, immunophenotype, genetics, and clinical features

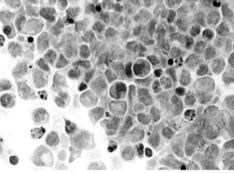

The appearance of AML

STAGING AND PROGNOSIS

- For adults there is an overall 25% five year survival
- Younger patients do much better than older patients

ACUTE MYELOID LEUKAEMIA

TREATMENT OPTIONS

- A multidisciplinary team approach is important
- Blood and/or platelet transfusions may be necessary
- Leukapheresis in those with a high leukocyte count (except for those that have acute promyelocytic leukaemia, due to the risk of bleeding)
- Chemotherapy is the primary treatment
- This is usually a very intense course that requires hospital admission (due to the intensity plus the high risk of tumour lysis syndrome, neutropenic sepsis and the likelihood of the need for symptom control)
- Initial 'induction' treatment usually includes cytarabine and daunorubicin

TREATMENT CONTINUED

- The follow on 'consolidation' treatment usually includes amsacrine, cytarabine and etoposide
- Growth colony simulating factors (GCSF) may be used for treating or preventing neutropenia or prior to a stem cell harvest
- Radiotherapy has a role either for cerebral spread or as total body irradiation prior to bone marrow transplantation
- Stem cell transplants to replace stem cells after high dose chemotherapy and/or total body irradiation can be autologous (cells are harvested from the patient themselves) or allogeneic (cells are harvested from either a close relative or an HLA matched unrelated donor)

ACUTE LYMPHOBLASTIC LEUKAEMIA

EPIDEMIOLOGY

- Overall, acute lymphoblastic leukaemia (ALL) is not as common as acute myeloid leukaemia (AML), but comprises 30% of all childhood malignancies (making it the most common childhood malignancy)
- There are around 600 new cases in the UK each year
- There is a peak of incidence between the ages of 2 and 5 and ALL is more common in boys than girls
- There is a smaller peak in adults aged over 50

RISK FACTORS INCLUDE

- Radiation exposure
- Benzene exposure
- Smoking or passive smoking for children
- Genetic conditions such as Down's syndrome, neurofibromatosis type 1, Fanconi's anaemla and ataxia telangiectasia
- There is a 25% concordance for monozygotic twins
- There is a four fold increase in risk if a dizygotic twin has ALL
- Previous chemotherapy drugs (particularly etoposide, mitoxantrone, amsacrine and idarubicin)
- Breastfed children and those that are exposed to common infections early such as at a nursery may have a slightly reduced risk

TYPES/PATHOLOGY/ SCREENING

- ALL is a haemopoietic malignancy involving precursor cells of the lymphoid line that are progenitors of B and T lymphocytes
- As with AML there are two different classifications; the French-American-British (FAB) system and the WHO system which is now more frequently used
- The FAB system divides ALL into three types:
  - L1 (most mature lymphocyte appearance)
  - L2
  - L3 (most immature lymphocyte appearance)
- The WHO system is based on the type of lymphocyte affected (B or T cell and either precursor or mature)
- Around 70% of cases are of the precursor B cell type
- Chromosomal abnormalities are common such as the t(9;22) BCR/ABL translocation (the Philadelphia chromosome), which is present in around 75% of ALL, particularly in older children
- There are also other cytogenetic abnormalities including
  - t(variable; 11q23), which is present in 60% of infant aged patients
  - t(12;21) ETV6/RUNX1, which is present in 25% of cases but is a good prognostic indicator

ACUTE LYMPHOBLASTIC LEUKAEMIA

SIGNS & SYMPTOMS

- Fatigue and malaise
- Recurrent fevers (often in the absence of infection)
- Frequent infections
- Bone pain, especially in long bones
- Lymphadenopathy
- Bleeding, bruising, petechiae and purpura
- Pallor
- Weight loss
- Headache
- Testicular mass
- Mediastinal mass (especially in adolescents)
- Dyspnoea
- Hepatomegaly
- Splenomegaly

INVESTIGATIONS

- An FBC will typically show significant anaemia, with a varying amount of thrombocytopenia and neutropenia
- A blood film may show blast cells
- Other blood tests including U&Es, LFTs, bone profile, clotting, urate, LDH and a viral screen
- Further tests for infection in patients with fever (blood cultures for example)
- Bone marrow aspirate and trephine biopsy
- Immunophenotyping (and HLA matching if a bone marrow transplant is a possibility)
- Cytogenetics
- Lumbar puncture
- A chest x-ray may show infection, a mediastinal mass or lytic bone lesions
- CT scan
- Testicular ultrasound scan
- Abdominal ultrasound scan

STAGING AND PROGNOSIS

- The overall five year survival rate for children is 85%
- But this falls to around 40% for adults
- The poorer outcome in adult patients is because they are more likely to have a cytogenetic abnormality
- Children under the age of 1 have a cure rate of just 30%
- Female patients tend to do better than males
- A high lymphocyte count at presentation is a poor prognostic indicator

TREATMENT OPTIONS

- A multidisciplinary team approach is important
- Blood and/or platelet transfusions may be necessary
- At diagnosis patients may require antibiotics for proven infection or correction of metabolic disturbances
- The mainstay of treatment is chemotherapy which is split into three stages
- The initial induction stage usually requires hospital admission for intensive chemotherapy, steroids and for some, radiotherapy
- Consolidation therapy involves further chemotherapy, often for around six months and possibly an allogeneic transplant
- Maintenance therapy then involves further, lower dose chemotherapy, for up to two years and short courses of steroids
- This prolonged maintenance stage is important as relapsed ALL has a very poor prognosis
- Growth factors and prophylaxis for tumour lysis syndrome (usually allopurinol) is given along with the chemotherapy
- Tyrosine kinase inhibitors can be used for Philadelphia chromosome positive ALL as part of the induction therapy

OTHER INTERESTING POINTS

- There are a number of complications that may arise due the toxicity of the chemotherapy agents used, which include
  - Infection, including neutropenic sepsis and opportunistic infections
  - Tumour lysis syndrome, particularly in children
  - Anaemia and bleeding
  - Hair loss
  - Gastrointestinal upset
  - Nephrotoxicity and hepatotoxicity
  - Peripheral neuropathy
  - Sinus venous thrombosis
  - Growth delay
  - Cardiomyopathy
  - Pulmonary fibrosis
  - Secondary malignancies
- Survival rates have dramatically improved since the 1980's and this is mainly thanks to the large number of children that have participated in research studies

CHRONIC MYELOID LEUKAEMIA

EPIDEMIOLOGY

- Chronic myeloid leukaemia (CML) accounts for around 15% of leukaemias
- It can occur at any age, but is rare in children (making up just 5% of childhood leukaemias) and is most common in those aged over 50
- There are around 600 new cases each year in the UK

RISK FACTORS INCLUDE

- The Philadelphia chromosome
- Radiation exposure
- Immunosuppression, particularly HIV
- Inflammatory bowel disease

SIGNS & SYMPTOMS

- Between a quarter and one half of patients are asymptomatic at diagnosis (made from a routine blood test)
- Fatigue
- Weight loss
- Night sweats
- Abdominal fullness
- Easy bleeding and bruising
- Splenomegaly
- Hepatomegaly
- Bone pain
- Patients may also present with gout or symptoms of hyperviscosity syndrome

TYPES/PATHOLOGY/ SCREENING

- CML is a myeloproliferative malignancy involving dysregulated production of mature and maturing granulocytes, particularly neutrophils, but also basophils and eosinophils
- A key part of CML is the t(9;22) BCR/ABL translocation (Philadelphia chromosome)
- The BCR/ABL gene codes for a fusion protein with deregulated (excessive) tyrosine kinase activity
- This cytogenetic abnormality is present in over 90% of cases of CML
- CML has a biphasic or triphasic clinical course; the initial chronic phase, progression to an accelerated phase and then a blast phase
- In up to a third of patients, the chronic phase moves directly into the blast phase

INVESTIGATIONS

- An FBC tends to show an anaemia with a significant leukocytosis
- Platelets should be normal or high
- Other blood tests including a blood film, U&Es, LFTs, bone profile, clotting, urate, LDH and a viral screen
- Bone marrow aspiration and trephine biopsy
- Cytogenetic analysis
- Tissue typing (HLA matching) if a stem cell transplant is a possibility
- Abdominal ultrasound

TREATMENT OPTIONS

- Treatment depends upon the phase of CML and performance status of the patient
- Imatinib (a tyrosine kinase inhibitor) is usually the first choice treatment in the chronic phase
- Nilotinib is also recommended by NICE as a first line treatment
- If the patient progresses to the accelerated phase the options include a switch to a different tyrosine kinase inhibitor, a trial of an older treatment such as interferon or hydroxyurea or alternatively a bone marrow or stem cell transplant
- In the blast phase the approach is similar to that of an acute leukaemia
- Cytotoxic agents can be used for palliation

STAGING AND PROGNOSIS

- Overall five year survival is 60%
- Those that are in the chronic phase and can tolerate a tyrosine kinase inhibitor can expect a five year survival of 89%

OTHER INTERESTING POINTS

- It is important to realise that even though tyrosine kinase inhibitors have revolutionised the treatment of CML, and whilst they can be taken as a tablet at home and have a mild side effect profile, they do not offer a cure, only control of the disease
- In more advanced disease, CML is less likely to be sensitive to imatinib, or resistance can develop relatively quickly
- Cell transplantation can offer a cure, but it is not without significant risks of morbidity and mortality

CHRONIC LYMPHOCYTIC LEUKAEMIA

EPIDEMIOLOGY

- Chronic lymphocytic leukaemia (CLL) is the most common form of leukaemia in western countries, making up around 30% of cases
- The incidence is very low in Asia and it is thought to be genetic rather than environmental factors that account for this
- The incidence increases with age; 75% are aged over 60 at diagnosis
- CLL is more common in males than females

RISK FACTORS INCLUDE

- Family history of CLL
- Interestingly, radiation exposure has not been shown to increase the risk of CLL, like it has for other forms of leukaemia

SIGNS & SYMPTOMS

- Between a quarter and one half of patients are asymptomatic at diagnosis (made from a routine blood test)
- Lymphadenopathy
- Splenomegaly
- Hepatomegaly
- Abdominal discomfort
- Bleeding, bruising or petechiae
- Fatigue
- Weight loss
- Fevers
- Night sweats
- Increased susceptibility to infections

TYPES/PATHOLOGY/ SCREENING

- CLL is a monoclonal expansion of B lymphocytes
- For a diagnosis to be made the absolute blood B lymphocyte count must exceed 5×10^9/L for three months and clonality should be demonstrated by flow cytometry
- Whilst CLL lymphocytes may appear mature, they are in fact developmentally and functionally immature and have three key immunophenotypic characteristics
  - The expression of CD19, CD20, and CD23 antigens
  - The expression of CD5, which is a T cell antigen
  - Low levels of surface membrane immunoglobulin

INVESTIGATIONS

- An FBC shows lymphocytosis and possibly anaemia
- Other blood tests including a blood film, U&Es, LFTs, bone profile, clotting, urate, LDH, immunoglobulins and a viral screen
- Direct Coombs' test
- Immunophenotyping
- Lymph node biopsy
- TP53 abnormality screening
- Bone marrow aspirate and cytogenetics are not always performed
- Chest x-ray and abdominal ultrasound scan

TREATMENT OPTIONS

- As CLL develops slowly and is typically a disease of the elderly, a watch and wait approach is often employed
- If however, there are signs of active disease chemotherapy is the treatment of choice
- Rituximab may be part of the treatment
- Steroids can be a useful part of a regime as they do not cause bone marrow suppression
- Allogeneic stem-cell transplantation should be considered as consolidation therapy for all fit patients with high risk CLL
- A splenectomy may be considered
- Radiotherapy is used palliatively for bulky node disease, splenomegaly or bone pain

STAGING AND PROGNOSIS

- The Binet staging system is used which is based upon clinical examination and blood tests rather than imaging
  - Stage A: Fewer than three lymph node sites involved with lymphocytosis but no anaemia or thrombocytopenia
  - Stage B: Three or more lymph node sites involved and lymphocytosis but no anaemia or thrombocytopenia
  - Stage C: Enlarged nodes or spleen and lymphocytosis with anaemia and/or thrombocytopenia
- Overall five year survival is 46%

OTHER INTERESTING POINTS

- Richter's syndrome (see lymphoma section) can occur and CLL can also transform into prolymphocytic leukaemia

MYELOMA

EPIDEMIOLOGY

- There are around 4600 new cases of myeloma each year in the UK
- It is more common in males and in Afro-Caribbean populations
- The incidence increases with age and 90% of diagnoses are in those aged over 50

RISK FACTORS INCLUDE

- Monoclonal gammopathy of unknown significance (MGUS)
- Family history of myeloma or MGUS
- Immunosuppression
- Being overweight

SIGNS & SYMPTOMS

- Bone pain
- Fatigue and lethargy
- Weight loss
- Dehydration
- Recurrent infections
- Bleeding and bruising
- Symptoms of hypercalcaemia (such as thirst, constipation, vomiting and confusion)
- Spinal cord or root compression

TYPES/PATHOLOGY/ SCREENING

- Myeloma is a malignant proliferation of bone marrow plasma cells producing a monoclonal immunoglobulin
- The immunoglobulin subclasses occur in the following order of frequency: IgG, IgA, light chain only, non-secretory, IgD, biclonal, IgM and IgE
- Light chains can precipitate in the renal tubules causing renal failure
- The main indication for treatment is evidence of end organ damage
- Myeloma is incurable

STAGING

- The international staging system is used:
- Stage 1: ß2-microglobulin <3.5mg/l and albumin >3.5g/dl
- Stage 2: ß2-microglobulin 3.5-5.5mg/l or albumin <3.5g/dl
- Stage 3: ß2-microglobulin >5.5mg/l

INVESTIGATIONS

- An FBC typically shows a normocytic, normochromic anaemia
- ESR is often significantly elevated
- Other blood tests, particularly looking at renal function, albumin, calcium and urate
- Immunoglobulin levels and electrophoresis
- Blood film (rouleaux formation)
- Free light chain assay (Freelite)
- ß2-microglobulin
- Urine protein electrophoresis (for Bence Jones protein)
- Bone marrow aspirate and trephine +/- cytogenetics
- Skeletal survey

TREATMENT OPTIONS

- Multidisciplinary approach
- High dose therapy (chemotherapy) with autologous stem cell transplantation is the recommended first line treatment for fit individuals
- Standard chemotherapy is most frequently the oral regime of cyclophosphamide, thalidomide and dexamethasone (CTD)
- Control of pain is important and may require a combination of NSAIDs, neuropathic painkillers, opiates, steroids, radiotherapy and bisphosphonates
- Bisphosphonates may also be used in an attempt to prevent fractures and for treatment of hypercalcaemia
- Biological therapies are available such as bortezomib (for people who can't take thalidomide) or lenalidomide (for those that have had previous treatment)
- Blood transfusions or plasmapheresis may be required

PROGNOSIS

- Overall five year survival is 37%
- For patients aged under 60 and fit enough for intensive treatment, five year survival is 50%

OTHER INTERESTING POINTS

- MGUS carries a risk of progression to myeloma of 1% per year
- A single lesion is known as a plasmacytoma, and a significant number of patients go on to develop myeloma

OTHER

POLYCYTHAEMIA VERA

- Polycythaemia vera (PV), a myeloproliferative disorder, is characterised by the clonal proliferation of myeloid cells leading to an elevated red blood cell mass
- There is also thrombocytosis and leukocytosis
- PV can occur in all ages and populations, although it is most common between the ages of 50 and 70
- The diagnosis may be made based on blood tests in asymptomatic individuals
- The most common presenting features are headache, dizziness, excessive sweating, aquagenic pruritus and erythromelalgia
- Around a quarter of patients present with an arterial or venous thrombotic event
- Patients may also experience transient visual disturbance and gastrointestinal symptoms
- Splenomegaly and hypertension are commonly found on examination
- Many patients have elevated leukocyte alkaline phosphatase and B12 levels and these are minor diagnostic criteria
- Around 98% of patients have a Janus kinase 2 (JAK2) mutation
- Management of PV involves venesection, prevention of thrombosis and in some cases cytoreduction
- With treatment, median survival is in excess of 10 years, but there is a significant risk of transformation to acute myeloid leukaemia

ESSENTIAL THROMBOCYTHAEMIA

- Essential thrombocythaemia is a chronic myeloproliferative disorder characterised by an overproduction of platelets
- A diagnosis can be made after reactive causes and other myeloproliferative disorders have been excluded
- It is extremely rare in children, but can occur at any adult age
- Around a half of patients are asymptomatic at presentation
- Signs and symptoms can include headache, dizziness, syncope, atypical chest pain, acral paraesthesia, livedo reticularis, moderate splenomegaly, thrombosis and haemorrhage
- Around 50% have a JAK2 mutation
- Treatment options include aspirin, chemotherapy and interferon
- Transformation to polycythaemia vera, myelofibrosis or acute leukaemia can occur

MYELOFIBROSIS

- Myelofibrosis is a chronic myeloproliferative disorder that is characterised by replacement of the bone marrow with fibrosis, which results in circulating immature cells of the granulocyte series, nucleated red cells and tear drop shaped poikilocytes
- The fibrosis is thought to be a result of growth factors produced by a high number of megakaryocytes
- It mainly affects the middle aged and elderly
- Signs and symptoms include fatigue, excessive sweating, weight loss, pruritus, arthralgia, splenomegaly, thrombotic events, pulmonary hypertension and hepatomegaly
- Anaemia is common, but platelet and leukocyte counts vary depending upon the stage of the condition (they are initially raised, but drop off later in the disease course as there is more fibrosis)
- Bone marrow aspiration usually results in a 'dry tap'
- 45-65% are JAK2 positive
- Treatment options are limited and focus upon correction of anaemia, control of leukocyte and platelet counts and control of constitutional symptoms
- Ruxolitinib, a Janus kinase inhibitor is showing promising results in those who are JAK2 positive
- Allogeneic stem cell transplantation is the only chance of cure but is high risk
- Transformation to an acute leukaemia can occur

MYELODYSPLASTIC SYNDROMES

- Myelodysplastic syndromes (MDS) are a group of clonal disorders resulting in peripheral blood cytopenias
- There is a high tendency for progression to acute myeloid leukaemia
- 80% of cases occur in those aged over 60
- Signs and symptoms are related to the cytopenias and include fatigue, recurrent or opportunistic infections and bleeding or bruising
- Treatment is largely supportive and can include red cell and platelet transfusions, erythropoietin and growth colony stimulating factor
- Haematopoietic stem cell transplantation is the only chance of cure, but is high risk and requires a matched donor
- Prognosis is poor

KEY POINTS SUMMARY

Hodgkin's lymphoma
- There are around 1500 new cases of Hodgkin's lymphoma each year in the UK
- Painless cervical or supraclavicular lymphadenopathy is the most common presenting sign
- The key to the diagnosis of Hodgkin's lymphoma is the presence of Reed-Sternberg cells
- With survival increasing, the incidence of secondary malignancies is important

Non-Hodgkin's lymphoma
- Non-Hodgkin's lymphoma is more than five times more common and more frequently disseminated at diagnosis than Hodgkin's lymphoma
- Chemotherapy is the primary treatment

Acute myeloid leukaemia
- Acute myeloid leukaemia is the most common acute leukaemia in adults
- An FBC will typically show a large number of blasts with depleted neutrophils, anaemia and thrombocytopenia
- Chemotherapy, initially as a very intensive course, is the primary treatment

Acute lymphoblastic leukaemia
- Acute lymphoblastic leukaemia the most common childhood malignancy
- The Philadelphia chromosome is present in around 75% of cases of ALL, particularly in older children
- The overall five year survival rate for children is 85%

Chronic myeloid leukaemia
- Chronic myeloid leukaemia accounts for around 15% of leukaemias and is rare in children
- The Philadelphia chromosome is present in around 90% of cases
- Tyrosine kinase inhibitors have revolutionised the treatment of CML

Chronic lymphoblastic leukaemia
- Chronic lymphocytic leukaemia is the most common form of leukaemia in western countries
- As CLL develops slowly and is typically a disease of the elderly, a watch and wait approach is often employed

Myeloma
- There are around 4600 new cases of myeloma each year in the UK, 90% of which are in those aged over 50
- Myeloma is a malignant proliferation of bone marrow plasma cells producing a monoclonal immunoglobulin
- MGUS carries a risk of progression to myeloma of 1% per year
- High dose chemotherapy with autologous stem cell transplantation is the recommended first line treatment for fit individuals

Others
- Polycythaemia vera is a myeloproliferative disorder characterised by the clonal proliferation of myeloid cells leading to an elevated red blood cell mass
- Essential thrombocythaemia is a chronic myeloproliferative disorder characterised by an overproduction of platelets
- Myelofibrosis is a chronic myeloproliferative disorder that is characterised by replacement of the bone marrow with fibrosis which results in circulating immature cells of the granulocyte series, nucleated red cells and tear drop shaped poikilocytes
- Myelodysplastic syndromes (MDS) are a group of clonal disorders resulting in peripheral blood cytopenias

ONCOLOGICAL EMERGANCIES

NEUTROPENIC SEPSIS

- Patients can deteriorate rapidly and die!
- Vigilance and a high index of suspicion is therefore vital
- The definition is neutrophils less than 1.0×10^9/L with septic symptoms
- The at risk 'nadir' period is classically between seven and fourteen days post chemotherapy due to bone marrow suppression
- Once neutrophils are below 0.5×10^9/L the risk of sepsis rapidly increases
- Additional risk factors include disruption of anatomical barriers and indwelling lines
- The usual signs of infection can often be absent in neutropenic patients
- Patients should be advised to check their temperature and report any increases (above 37.5°C on two occasions separated by at least one hour or one occasion above 38.5°C)
- If neutropenic sepsis is suspected, IV access should be obtained, blood taken including FBC and cultures and then broad spectrum antibiotics and intravenous fluids administered
- There should be a 'door to needle' time of under an hour
- Further investigations include chest x-ray, urine dipstick and culture, cultures and swabs from any lines, skin and throat swabs and stool and sputum cultures as appropriate
- The patient should be examined with a focus on potential foci for infection and haemodynamic status
- PR examination should not be performed on neutropenic patients
- Consideration should be given to administering anti-fungal or antiviral therapy
- Further management is similar to that of management of sepsis in other circumstances
- Intravenous antibiotics should be continued until patient is apyrexial and the neutrophil count is above 0.5×10^9/L and rising
- After this point, if a source has been identified, antibiotics can be stepped down to a narrower spectrum and/or oral alternative
- If the patient continues to spike a temperature beyond 48 hours antibiotics should be switched to the second line choice and further thought given to atypical, fungal and viral infections
- In persistently neutropenic, granulocyte colony stimulating factor can improve the rate of recovery
- It is appropriate to consider resuscitation status after the initial assessment and discussion with patient and/or family

SPINAL CORD COMPRESSION

- Occurs in around 5% of patients with cancer
- It's most commonly associated with myeloma and prostate cancer (but also breast, lung, non-Hodgkin's lymphoma and renal cancers)
- 23% of patients diagnosed with spinal metastasis have not previously been given a cancer diagnosis
- The main mechanism is extradural metastases causing compression (in at least 80% of cases)
- Intradural compression from a primary spinal cord tumour or secondary deposit can also occur
- 70% occur in the thoracic spine due to the shape of the vertebrae, 20% in the lumbar spine and 10% in the cervical spine
- 20% will have compression at more than one site
- The earliest symptom is vertebral pain especially on coughing and lying flat
- Other signs and symptoms include radicular pain, leg weakness, increased reflexes, urinary dysfunction, constipation and a sensory level
- Discordance between the symptoms and level of compression is common
- The key investigation is MRI of the whole spine
- Initial management is strict bed rest, administration of steroids, usually 8mg of dexamethasone, followed by 16mg daily in two or four divided doses with gastric protection
- Analgesia is usually also required
- The patient should then be discussed as appropriate with a clinical oncologist or spinal surgeon, although most hospitals now have a spinal cord compression co-ordinator
- Surgery is usually preferred as it offers a more rapid decompression and also provides the opportunity to obtain histology in patients whose cause is unknown
- However, patients that are not fit enough to have surgery, have multiple levels of compression, have a radiosensitive tumour, have a life expectancy of less than three months or do not want to have surgery are offered radiotherapy as an alternative
- Realistically, full recovery can only be expected if the symptoms are of less than 24 hours duration and the neurological loss is not complete at the time of treatment
- As such it is important to have a high index of suspicion for spinal cord compression to prevent the consequences of a delayed diagnosis

ONCOLOGICAL EMERGANCIES

SUPERIOR VENA CAVA OBSTRUCTION

- Superior vena cava obstruction (SVCO) can be caused by external compression or obstruction or thrombosis of the vessel
- At least 70% of cases are due to lung cancers
- Other causes include lymphoma, nodal metastases, germ cell tumours and malignant or non-malignant lymphadenopathy
- Signs and symptoms include dyspnoea, neck, face and arm oedema, dizziness, headache, disturbed vision, dilated veins in the distribution of the vessel and stridor
- Patients may also present with cough and chest pain, but these are more likely due to the underlying tumour
- Investigations include chest x-ray (may be normal), lymph node biopsy, doppler scan and CT thorax
- Immediate management includes oxygen, elevation of the head, steroids and diuretics
- Further management is focused on the underlying cause and may include radiotherapy, chemotherapy or anticoagulation
- If SVCO is recurrent or non-responsive to treatment a stent should be considered

HYPERCALCAEMIA

- Hypercalcaemia affects up to 25% of cancer patients
- It is most common in myeloma, breast, lung and renal cancers and T cell lymphoma
- Bony metastasis are absent in 20% of cases
- The main causes are bone metastases, PTH related peptide secretion by the tumour, dehydration and drugs (such as thiazides and tamoxifen)
- Symptoms include nausea, vomiting, fatigue, thirst, polyuria, muscle weakness, confusion, constipation and abdominal pain
- Investigations include measurement of adjusted calcium, ALP and PTH, x-rays and a bone scan
- Initial management is with normal saline which increases renal excretion of calcium and rehydrates the patient
- If the patient is or becomes fluid overloaded concurrent furosemide can be administered
- Intravenous bisphosphonates can be given after rehydration (but there is a delay in action)
- Further management involves addressing the underlying malignancy if possible
- 30 day mortality is almost 50%

TUMOUR LYSIS SYNDROME

- The metabolic disturbance of hyperkalaemia, hyperphosphataemia, hyperuricaemia and hypocalcaemia that can lead to acute kidney injury and cardiac arrhythmias
- Tumour lysis syndrome is associated with treatment sensitive cancers such as acute leukaemias, high grade lymphoma and some solid tumours
- Patients who are at high risk are often given preventative treatment such as intravenous fluids and rasburicase or allopurinol
- Onset is usually within 72 hours of treatment
- Investigations in suspected cases includes FBC, biochemistry, urine output measuring and pH and cardiac monitoring
- Initial treatment is aggressive hydration to maintain good urine output and correction of the metabolic disturbances, particularly the hyperkalaemia
- Rasburicase or allopurinol can be administered for the hyperuricaemia
- Hypocalcaemia in the presence of hyperphosphataemia should only be corrected if symptomatic due to the risk of precipitation of calcium phosphate
- Dialysis may be needed in some cases

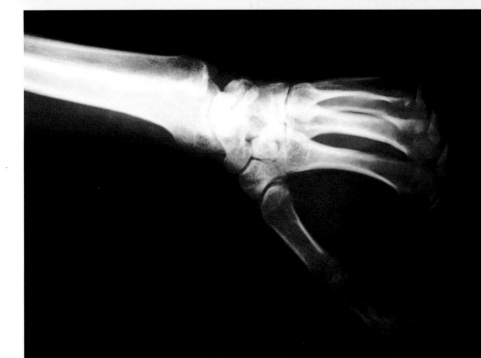

RHEUMATOLOGY

FOR MEDICAL STUDENTS AND JUNIOR DOCTORS

2nd Edition

Dr Matthew Langtree

LESS TIME, MORE KNOWLEDGE